STRESS AND ADAPTATION
IN PHYSIOLOGY:

Perturbation - Between Poison and Medication

Cristian Vlad Zot

Page left blank intentionally

Note to the reader (disclaimer)

The information from this book is intended to explore the concepts of stress and adaptation. Do not use this book as a substitute for professional medical care or treatment.

Every effort has been made to ensure that the information contained in the book is complete and accurate. However, the author is not engaged in rendering advice to the individual reader.

This book should not serve as a how-to guide for any medical practice. If you decide to follow such endeavors, do it under the supervision of a qualified physician.

Table of Contents

Stress and Adaptation in Physiology

Introduction

Distant times and myth take us into to Kingdom of Pontus, a territory of Persian and Greek origins. Here, we meet a young boy, Mithridates VI Eupator, whose father had just been assassinated by poisoning.

It was the year 120 B.C., and the half-formed Mithridates painfully accepted that running away into wilderness was the best way to escape the auspices of his mother, Laodice VI. She unlawfully claimed the throne together with Mithridates' younger brother.

Several years have passed until Mithridates came out of his hiding. Removing his mother and brother from reign, he imprisoned them. He was hailed king and he ruled until 63 B.C.

He did not have an easy going as king. A fearless leader, Mithridates fought numerous battles, always seeking to expand the Pontic kingdom. This increasing power of his and the far-reaching territory brought together a growing number of enemies.

His alleged friends proved to be not so friendly after all. A few plotted against him, trying to murder him by poison, same as it happened with his father. Catching on these plots early, Mithridates not only killed them, but their families as well.

One of his sons, his own flesh and blood, led a rebellion against him. In 63 B.C., Mithridates was forced to withdraw from the kingdom. He thought he could plan a spontaneous comeback, but he wasn't able to gather sufficient military power.

Mithridates attempted suicide by poison. But, to his surprise, the substance he used had no effect. He was immune to it, so to speak. Thus, he ordered his Gaulish bodyguard to kill him by the sword (a much more certain approach!).

But why would Mithridates be immune to poison?

The assassination of his father led him to suspect his mother's involvement into the ordeal. He then remembered that while still at the throne, his father often complained about stomach pains during meals. Mithridates reasoned that his mother ordered a slow death for the king by adding poisonous substances to his food. Thinking that he would be the next in line, Mithridates fled into the wild soon after the death of his father.

Of course, he was not to live as an outcast forever. He had to figure out something that would protect him against such plots and attacks. The time will come for him to reclaim the throne, he reasoned. He had to be prepared.

Mithridates was about 13 years old when his father died. It is said that while maturing in the wild he subjected himself to hardship. He developed immunity by regular self-administration of sub-lethal doses of poison:

"...to secure her own position, she tried to do away with Eupator: the boy's guardians, we are told, forced him to ride and throw the javelin from a dangerous horse, and when this failed to kill him, they turned to the surer means of poison. He was on his guard, however, and took antidotes to buildup an immunity, which worked so effectively that he was unable to kill himself by poison at the end of his reign.

To avoid these attempts on his life Eupator removed himself from the court and lived in the woods, where he grew strong by hunting, and became used to all hardship." [1]

His universal antidote contained a few dozen ingredients that were to be placed in a flask and left to mature for at least 60 days. For this practice, Mithridates VI Eupator was to be known and remembered as the father of *mithridatism*, which is the act of self-administering sub-lethal doses *of the same* (substance, I assume) to protect oneself against more severe poisoning.

Poisonous tree extracts, venom and other *natural* toxins may elicit immunity enhancing effects, while base chemicals, man made toxic substances and other synthetic compounds may have no effects, and could be detrimental in certain situations.

The argument that the toxic effects of synthetic chemicals are experienced at all doses is still debated because stress physiology, dose response relationships, and something called *hormesis*, have been receiving increased attention from the scientific community lately.

Putting aside mythical stories and times immemorial, let us explore these matters by modern day account.

Stress and adaptation is the main subject of this book. Numerous current studies overcomplicate these mechanisms by using them in sophisticated terminology.

One of such terms is *hormesis*. I will use this term here and there, throughout the book, mainly because it was found in the literature that I cite. My point is, however, not to propose, promote, or support hormesis (in fact, I don't like this term - subjectively speaking), but to provide a deeper understanding of stress and adaptation.

A large part of the existing literature (scientific and popular) on stress is focused on psychology, personal motivation, and other topics different from physiology. Thus, one of my main reasons for writing this book was to explore and provide a current perspective on stress and adaptation in physiology.

In the following pages, I make the distinction between hormesis, homeostasis, and homeopathy, which are often confused with one another. For introductory purposes though, I feel the need to outline a simple view of hormesis provided by two of its proponents.

From Mattson and Calabrese's textbook (2009), we learn that hormesis *"describes any process in which a cell, organism, or group of organisms exhibits a biphasic response to exposure to increasing amounts of a substance or condition."* [2]

The definition may seem straightforward even to the lay person, except for the use of the term 'biphasic', which refers to the dual nature of the response. Plainly, hormesis is characterized by a biphasic dose response curve in the following way; it can elicit:

- beneficial (stimulatory, positive) responses at low-dose exposure to the stressor.
- detrimental (inhibitory, toxic) responses at high-dose exposure to the stressor.

Examples of such stressors can be: metabolic, environmental, toxic substances, sensory, nutritional, etc. Thus, more elegantly and more concisely put, hormesis refers to:

A process in which exposure to a low dose of a chemical agent or environmental factor, that is damaging at higher doses, induces an adaptive beneficial effect on the cell or organism. [2]

Both evidence-based and anecdotal connections have been ascribed to hormesis. Some of them refer to:

- positive effects from low-dose exposure to food toxins
- how timed resistance training builds muscle, while too much/heavy/prolonged/chronic resistance training may have a detrimental effect
- how free radicals can have a positive impact on physiology

- how fasting, intermittent fasting, and other dietary restriction protocols promote autophagy and can build resilience, while starvation and malnutrition may be slippery slopes to ill health
- how acute cold and heat stress can build resilience, while prolonged exposure to extreme temperatures can be lethal
- how radiation can be beneficial
- and so on.

All of these topics, and a few more, represent the subject of this book. Each of them will be treated with the appropriate level of detail. With my current knowledge, I will try to draw a critical perspective from the research studies mentioned in the book. The anecdotal evidence I use comes from my personal experiments with each of these protocols. I consider both evidence and anecdote important for the sake of superior understanding of stress and adaptation.

Not having personal experience on the subject matter, I would not be able to understand the research literature and I would not be able to see the practicality and applicability of the subject matter. Having only personal experience, without the scientific understanding of the topic, would prevent me from deriving meaningful insights that could potentially be helpful for others too.

Hence, my purpose with this book is to help both you and I to make better, more critical, and more informed choices, should we decide to follow strategies for coping with physiologic stress. Let me briefly provide a couple of anecdotal examples.

I am sure you know:

- a person who religiously follows a certain diet and does not want to touch a piece of the forbidden food; the person who *can* only consume food that is gluten free, organically grown, sugar free, or any other food labeled with the word 'free' on it.

- a person who needs to go to the gym 7 days a week, otherwise they will lose the 'gains'.

- a person who fears the chemicals in soaps, plastics, and those found in beauty products; or the person who fears food 'toxins', whatever the meaning of that term is.

And in the most extreme of cases, you probably know someone who meets all these criteria. Judging only by the dietary aspects and the dietary phobias, if I may, this person could be called an orthorexic.

Sanchez and colleagues (2005) [3] explain that *orthorexia* is characterized by a pathologic obsession for consuming biologically pure foods only, and that orthorexics (people who suffer from orthorexia) exclude foods they consider impure because of their minute contents of pesticides, herbicides, and artificial substances.

Similarly, *bigorexia*, a new word with recent high circulation in the media, alludes to muscle dysmorphia and the obsession of being too *small* (in terms of muscle mass). It will be interesting to explore both of these terms in the context of positive physiologic stress.

Another example relevant to the potential benefits of appropriate exposure to stressors is when you compare the physical appearance of a marathon runner to that of a sprinter (short-distance runner). While one is chronically exposed to the stimulus (running) for long periods of time (marathoner), the other one gets short, but extremely intense, bouts of the stimulus (sprinter). If you use your preferred search engine to find images of sprinters and marathoners, you could notice the difference.

I want to point out that extremes like these (orthorexia, prolonged chronic exercise, bigorexia, prolonged temperature stress, prolonged radiation exposure, etc.) may not be beneficial. This is when too much of a stressor becomes a problem. While taking something to the extremes for a short period of time (acute stress) can situationally elicit positive effects, chronic stress, more often than not, leads to negative effects.

Alluding to the psychologic aspects of stressors, staying average and not moving outside the boundaries of your comfort zone (lack of stress) is not good either. It increases fragility (vulnerability), it does not help one grow (in any aspect) and it, most likely, *leads to a mediocre life*.

Thus, it becomes challenging to find an appropriate level of stress and stressors to be administered at an appropriate frequency, and duration of exposure to lead to positive adaptations. My objective with this book is to discuss positive acute stress (eustress) applied contextually (fasting, radiation, exercise, plant toxins, etc).

With the risk of appearing too boring, I have to start by presenting the modern-day perspective of the subject matter, introducing terms like hormesis, homeostasis and homeopathy, and the potential scientific evidence or lack thereof to support them.

As we go through the book and as the concepts become clearer, I will propose practical applications of physiologic stress in daily life. Lastly, I will associate stressors with the concept of *anti-fragility* by deriving insights and by building upon the work of Nassim Nicholas Taleb (risk analyst, essayist, and statistician).

When it comes to my personal approach, there have been a couple of experiments that have to do with deliberate exposure to stressor. I applied this concept within the contexts of: cold and heat exposure, intermittent and prolonged fasting, use of dietary phytochemicals, resistance training, supplementation, ketosis, and a few more.

Some of them have been discussed in my previous books, but I will provide an updated perspective here. One of my experiments, for which I did not provide enough detail (so far), involves temperature stress. Let me give you a brief context.

I started practicing cold exposure in the winter of 2012. I read an article on *gettingstronger.org* about its potential benefits [4]. When I began doing it, it was very intense. I was not used to deliberately taking myself out of my comfort zone. My cold exposure experiments would allow me to travel through time to my childhood when, during mountain trips, my father used to bathe in the nearly frozen river that ran by our tent. And, like father like son, I did just about the same thing. Those short cold plunges were so invigorating...

All those memories came back naturally when I started taking cold showers in late 2012. But now I was a young adult. And it was different. Between that moment and my childhood there was little to no experience with deliberately exposing myself to acute cold stress.

I can still remember the shyness of entering into the shower, slowly turning the shower knob to the neutral point (where cold and warm water meet), rationalizing what I was about to do. In fact, I wrote about the entire experience on my blog. Here's an excerpt from that post [5]:

"I was standing naked in front of the shower deciding whether I should do it or not. Ok, here goes!

I turned on the shower knob, half-way between the warm and cold water (at the mid-point). The water was quite cold, but I could tolerate it. It was beginning to become weird because I practically never did this before.

It took 15 seconds until I gradually shifted the knob to the extreme point of the cold water. Now I could feel the avalanche of cold coming to me. That's when things really started to become crazy. In the summer time here, if I want to take a cold shower, the tap water is not very cold because the pipelines are not buried deep in the ground and the heat from the outside raises the water temperature.

However, the same process takes place in the winter time because as the temperature outside gets colder, the tap water becomes extremely colder as well.

So, there I was. In shock! I felt and actually had my breath taken for a few seconds. This is known as the cold shock. The water was unbearably ice-cold.

*I started breathing faster and faster (hyperventilating). I felt how my body starts generating heat (this is actually the beginning of the process when your body burns fat to warm itself – **thermogenesis**).*

I was constantly changing the direction of the water, from my legs to my stomach, to my chest, to both of my arms, to the back of my neck, and eventually above my head. I couldn't keep it fixated for long.

The sensation was amazing. Something actually happened because I started feeling very well and after 20-30 seconds have passed and I was under the coldest water possible, my body started to get accommodated to it.

The whole extreme experience lasted for no more than 2 minutes. Some parts of my skin turned red due to the water temperature :). But it was a great feeling. It gave me a sensation of pure happiness. I knew that I would stick to that feeling."

As it turns out, there is a vast scientific literature regarding the impact of cold thermogenesis on human health. The challenge is, however, to filter through all the bad data (poorly conducted studies, authors with conflicting interests, studies supported by entities with some stake in the business, trivial/anecdotal data, and so on) and uncover whatever *good* science there is - from which practical and useful applications can be derived. Let's add this burdensome process of literature review to the repertoire of things I want to accomplish in this book.

In the chapter on temperature stress I also address heat exposure and the potential implications of heat shock proteins in human health.

Exposure to low-dose stressors that can lead to positive adaptations have also been reported in nutrition science. Fasting, either intermittently or prolonged, is considered by some researchers to be a forgotten evolutionary mechanism that allowed our early ancestors to survive during food shortage. Today, though, there rarely is such a shortage...

Here is a personal and anecdotal rant:

Look at where we are today as we cram our faces with food multiple times a day, 7 days a week, without ever even considering taking a break, *injecting* some randomness (strategic fasting) into such a fixated and fragile habit. We panic about a so called *starvation mode* when food is not ingested every few hours. (end of rant)

Starvation, a real medical phenomenon, mostly never occurs today. In one of my earlier books, *Periodic Fasting*, I described starvation as the process of breaking down muscle tissue to survive when bodyfat is so low that your metabolism can no longer use fat for energy [6]. When does that happen, you may wonder?

For example, a lean person, like me, who is about 174 cm tall (5 feet 9 inches), 65 kg (143 pounds) could undergo a couple of weeks of water only fasting (consuming nothing but water) until reaching the critically low bodyfat where starvation mode initiates (I assume other health parameters would be optimal during the fast).

Everything up to that point should be considered fasting and should not require association with dramatic words such as *starvation*.

Talking to someone who practiced prolonged water fasting and they would most likely report effects that include: increased physiologic and cognitive performance, alertness, and reduced or total lack of hunger. In most cases, hunger is gone after the first 1-2 days of water fasting, a transition period during which glycogen (stored glucose) is being depleted and the body shifts to predominantly using fat for energy.

If a lean person could safely undergo a couple of weeks of water fasting, then, the next logical question should be: how long could an overweight or obese person last on bodyfat and water alone?

Academia, medical journals and even the non-fiction literature (books) provide countless examples of people fasting (water only) for dozens and up to hundreds of days. The longest medically recorded fast lasted for 382 days (yes, more than a year). In this voluntary experiment entered a 200 kg (456 lb) Angus Barbieri and came out an 82 kg (180 lb) version of the same person [6]. Five years after the fast and Angus Babieri's weight remained stable at around 88 kg (196 lb).

The information and the data are all there, but they never spread into the mainstream because who would make money telling you not to buy this weight loss pill or that powder, but to consume nothing except water?! Fasting is unpopular and labeled as potentially dangerous. Our world is focused on massive consumption (food) and pill-popping. Very few, if any, supplements have a solid track record to efficiently support the process of weight loss.

Leaving the topic of water fasting aside for now, (well get into some more details later), intermittent fasting is a similar, shorter, more convenient, and often so very enjoyable meal timing strategy. It does not necessarily have to involve caloric restriction.

The most basic protocol of intermittent fasting (IF) is the 16-8 cycle, where you fast for at least 16 hours a day (fasting window), and you consume all your food in an 8-hour feeding window. The beauty of it is that it has shown benefits independent of caloric restriction. One only has to limit the timing of food intake to a certain feeding window everyday, without necessary limiting caloric intake.

Other, more advanced, IF protocols, discussed in my book *Persistent Fat Loss*, propose for longer fasting windows and shorter feeding windows. Two examples are IF 18-6 (18 hours of fasting, 6 hours of eating) and IF 20-4 (20 hours of fasting, 4 hours of eating).

With these advanced protocols the *challenge* of eating to maintenance becomes even harder because it is not easy to consume your day's worth of calories in a 6-hour (IF 18-6), 4-hour (IF 20-4) or even shorter feeding window. However, you can imagine the increase in satisfaction and satiety when consuming so much food in such a short time frame. Some people who practice daily IF also reduce caloric intake naturally, without shortage in satisfaction and satiety. I happen to be one of them.

Later in the book I'll expand on some of the details of water fasting and intermittent fasting and I'll explore adaptive mechanisms associated with these nutritional strategies. This may encourage you to add either one or both into your toolbox for improving your physiology.

Not leaving the nutrition field, I'll also explore the potential stressors that are present in food compounds. These are toxic food constituents that when consumed at low to moderate doses can provide positive adaptive health effects, while after a certain threshold (at higher doses), they may be detrimental to health. Most of these stressors are found in plant foods. Here, I'll also investigate the efficacy of supplementing with such compounds.

Orthorexia, the maniacal obsession with consuming only the purest of foods, will receive its attention in this part of the book too.

I want to discuss orthorexia and other food psychopathologies because I know that many people try to do everything the right way (when it comes to weight loss, muscle gain, alleviating/curing diseases, and so on) and they fail.

Genetics and epigenetics can shed some light on orthorexia. Exploring your genetics can play an important role to choosing an appropriate approach to health because the thousands of single nucleotide polymorphisms (SNPs) that are present in your genome make you unique in terms of susceptibility to certain physiologic and psychologic conditions.

This is one of the reasons I think that personalized health approaches make sense (instead of using general dietary/non-dietary guidelines). What's healthy for you could be poisonous for me. I could have a genetic mutation that makes me unable to process a certain food substance the same way as you do. I envision the coming of age of nutritional genomics. Long-gone are the days when everyone should follow a generalized dietary protocol: high-fat, low-fat, no fat, or everything in between.

Yet, genetics 'is' not everything; epigenetics also play an important role in health and disease. Regardless of the mutations you may have, you can impact the way your genes are expressed or silenced. It is not a death sentence if you carry a mutation in a gene involved in cancer development (say BRCA for example) if you implement lifestyle interventions to drastically reduce your risk for developing the disease - through good nutrition and exercise, to name only two.

In another chapter I will explore physical exercise, seeking appropriate doses to induce positive physiologic adaptations (muscle growth, better endurance, etc). Similar to nutrition, the science literature on physical exercise can be conflicting, and in order to derive practical insight from it, one requires knowledge of statistics, biochemistry, physiology and, more importantly, critical thinking skills.

Some say that to build muscle you have to exercise more frequently using lighter weights. These folks cite studies to prove their point). Others swear by drastically reducing frequency and significantly increasing intensity. They also use studies to rationalize their point. So, who is right and who is wrong?

Unsurprisingly, regardless of the quality of the studies cited, both strategies can prove correct, as long as a bigger picture is always in mind - where you acknowledge the implications of genetics, epigenetics, and other factors and where you try to control for as many variables as possible.

Radiation biology is another topic that I will address in the context of stress and adaptation. In fact, this is the field in which phenomena such as *hormesis* have been mostly explored from a research perspective.

If hormesis proves to be a solid and widely-applicable mechanism, I think it will be challenging to find appropriate doses for each *hormetic* stressor to yield the desired positive adaptation. Context-based and individualized strategies will be paramount.

With that in mind...

We are almost always exposed to different levels of different stressors - physiologic and psychologic perturbations. To simplistically approach positive adaptive stress by acutely increasing the exposure to a certain stressor can be dangerous. Think about it, for example:

It may be unreasonable for a sick or unhealthy person to expect positive health adaptations from jumping into ice cold water or from fasting for several days, without being somewhat preconditioned to such stressors. This would be reckless, to say the least. The vulnerable condition of the person and the very high level of acute stress (stressor) could make this experience a life-threatening one.

I will propose using a rational approach that focuses on gradually building tolerance for positive adaptations to occur. As one develops tolerance to a certain dose of a certain stressor, it can become challenging to maintain such positive health effects. This could be a call for a resensitization period, where one would deprive oneself of the stressor so that they can later reintroduce the exposure, using a much lower dose of the stressor.

Always changing the approach, the frequency of exposure, and the dose are critical for reaping the benefits of positive adaptive physiologic stress over the long run.

Flexibility reduces fragility. Seeking a fixated protocol for wellbeing (diet, exercise, cognitive performance, etc) to follow for the rest of your life will most likely make you vulnerable to non-compliance (falling off the wagon).

I know it all seems very abstract and unspecific for now, but I'm confident that you will understand my point as I provide examples and as I become more specific later in the book.

Looks like there's a lot ahead...

To grasp it all, we should first get a good hold of some terminology. I will start with an exploration of dose response relationships and biologic stress.

Date:
March 4, 2016

Chapter 1
Dose Response Relationships: An Intro

All things are poison and nothing is without poison, only the dose permits something not to be poisonous.

Paracelsus

Hormesis - a process characterized by a biphasic dose response of a cell or organism to a perturbing agent:

- low-dose exposure => stimulatory/beneficial effects (non-neutral)
- high-dose exposure => inhibitory/toxic effects.

This type of dose-response relationship has been described under several names across modern scientific research. However, in the past few years, it seems as though *hormesis* became the go-to term for this kind of effect.

As explained by Mattson and Calabrese (2009) [2], the response of the cell/organism to a low-dose exposure to a toxic/perturbing agent (stressor) involves disruption in **homeostasis**, which is then followed by an adaptive compensatory effect.

Homeostasis, in humans, is *"the maintenance of metabolic equilibrium by a tendency to compensate for disrupting changes"* [7]. Simply put, an organism always gravitates toward physiologic and metabolic equilibrium. This normal state of the body (homeostasis) is best understood with a few examples:

- keeping body temperature stable at ~36.7°C by sweating in excessive heat and by shivering when it gets too cold
- keeping blood glucose levels stable by regulating the secretion of insulin and glucagon
- keeping blood pH stable at 7.4

- keeping water content in the blood stable by extracting water from the cells, thus increasing it when the concentration gets too low, and by increasing diuresis (increasing urine production and excretion) when the concentration is too high
- regulating the number of cells so that organ/tissue size and function are stable
- restoring normal blood oxygen content when CO_2 concentration increases by increasing blood flow, heart beats, and depth and speed of breathing.

Thus, homeostasis describes an internal state of equilibrium (chemical balance); homeostatic mechanisms have the purpose of restoring this balance when perturbing factors deregulate it.

As of such, hormesis could be seen as factor to perturb homeostasis. If administered at an appropriate dose, the hormetic factor/stressor (often known as hormetin) may lead to positive adaptive changes as homeostasis is being restored within the biologic system.

Homeostasis receives appropriate scientific attention in most biochemistry textbook, while hormesis, not as pervasive, has mostly been described (so far) in toxicology related literature. And now, let's briefly move to less scientific concepts, such as homeopathy.

Hormesis is often confused with homeopathy; the only thing relating these two terms is probably their similarity in name.

Homeopathy is, according to Merriam Webster (2016), a system of medical practice treating diseases by *"the administration of minute doses of a remedy that in large quantities would produce in healthy persons symptoms similar to those of the disease"* [9]. I find it difficult to grasp the definition. Let's see how homeopathy practitioners and promoters describe their practice.

According to The Society of Homeopaths (2016), homeopathy *"involves treating the individual with highly diluted substances, given mainly in tablet form, with the aim of triggering the body's natural system of healing"* [10]. It was created in 1796 by Samuel Hahnemann based on his belief that *like cures like*:

"a substance which causes symptoms when taken in large doses, can be used in small amounts to treat similar symptoms." [10]

By 'small' they mean almost nonexistent. The high dilution they talk about makes some skeptics associate homeopathic dilutions with pure water, where almost no amount of the homeopathic substance is present. This makes me question the effectiveness of a solution that is, say, 3 parts per million (ppm) or 999,997 molecules of water (or any other dilute) and 3 molecules of the homeopathic substance.

Some critics are not so tolerant. They put it more bluntly, saying that homeopathy is pseudoscience (a claim, practice, or belief that is incorrectly presented as being scientific) and that homeopathic preparations are not effective in treating pathologic conditions or any health conditions for that matter [11] [12] [13] [14].

Large scale studies and reputable publications have found that homeopathy is no better than placebo. These studies suggest that any positive outcomes from homeopathy studies are due to the placebo effect and normal recovery from disease [15] [16] [17]. Often, placebo works better than homeopathy.

Placebo studies involve treating subjects with inert sugar pills or other inert (without effect) interventions. Subjects are told that the administration of such pills may improve their pathologic conditions. They are completely unaware of the inertness of the intervention, especially when the study is double-blind and randomized.

Often times, researchers see positive results from such interventions and they attribute these results to the subject's expectations from the intervention. If a subject expects a pill or anyother intervention to have an effect on their body, it is possible that auto-suggestion causes the effect that would normally be expected from a given medication or intervention.

Even though the research community uses the placebo effect at length, its exact mechanisms of action are not yet elucidated; suggestibility (self or non-self) is thought to play an important role.

Randomized, double blind, placebo controlled trials represent gold standards of research. They are some of the most favorite tools in evidence and science based medicine. However, it is not always possible to design and conduct such studies to test different hypotheses - mostly due to unpractical and unethical reasons.

Finding that homeopathy is no better than placebo (sometimes it is worse) is a big NO for this practice and it strengthens the general belief that homeopathy is a pseudoscience. That is why I will not devote paper space to discuss homeopathy in this book.

Hormesis may receive more scientific credit but its association (in name) with homeopathy may have diluted (if I may) this effect. Hormesis, despite its higher prevalence and validity, is still not something with strong scientific approval, even though some of its proponents may like to think so.

While I think that the mechanisms of hormesis seem to come from a rational approach in some circumstances, I do not agree with its proponents who claim that hormesis is a generalized mechanism. In my view, it is contextual, at most.

The strategies that I am going to discuss in this book involve strategically subjecting oneself to adversity and stress. This type of stress is positive, also known as eustress, and it can lead to beneficial physiologic and psychologic adaptations, if it is administered at an appropriate dose, frequency and timeliness.

I will allude to hormesis in certain parts of the book; thus, I find it obligatory to introduce some of its proponents and their ideas, as well as some of the critiques brought to this mechanism.

Contemporary Researchers of Hormesis

If you search the science literature for hormesis, you will most likely encounter a lot of papers written by Mark P. Mattson, Edward Calabrese, and Suresh Rattan to name a few. Often you will find papers written by these researchers in collaboration.

Mark Mattson, Ph.D., is currently the Chief of Laboratory of Neurosciences at the National Institute on Aging, Intramural Research Program. He also teaches in the Department of Neurosciences at Johns Hopkins University School of Medicine [18]. As a researcher, Mattson's activity is nothing short of extraordinary.

His full CV from 2014 is 81 pages long and lists 575 articles from peer reviewed journals that had his name on them. According to Google Scholar's profile of Mark Mattson, his papers have been cited for more than 100,000 times (officially) and his h-index (a measure of impact among researchers) is, as of 2016, 177, putting him among one of the most active and reputable contemporary scientists [19].

Mattson's main work involves understanding the mechanisms of brain aging as well as how neurodegenerative disorders emerge. He is also the editor of 19 books (as of 2014), most of them in the field of neuroscience and aging. We will derive a lot of insight from Mattson's overwhelming work throughout this book [18].

Edward Calabrese, Ph.D., is another scientist whose work I will mention. He is a Professor and the Program Director of Environmental Health Science at the University of Massachusetts, Amherst. According to his faculty page, his research focuses on environmental toxicology and host factors affecting susceptibility to pollutants [20].

Dr. Calabrese is the leading proponent in the area of radiation hormesis and he is, so very often, the go-to authority for this subject. Among other awards, in 2009, he received the Marie Curie Prize for his work on hormesis. Calabrese is the author and editor of more than 10 books. His full CV from 2013 is 145 pages long and he is the author of more than 750 papers published in scholarly journals [20] [21].

Over the past 20 years, Calabrese's research career has focused on understanding how low-dose responses to different stimuli can lead to positive adaptive mechanisms. Most importantly, he has provided arguments that mark a clear distinction between hormesis and homeopathy [20]:

"Of particular note is that this research has led to important discoveries which indicate that the most fundamental dose response in toxicology and pharmacology is the hormetic-biphasic dose response relationship. These observations are leading to a major transformation in improving drug discovery, development, and in the efficiency of the clinical trial, as well as the scientific foundations for risk assessment and environmental regulation for radiation and chemicals."

Since 2014, Calabrese has been an Adjunct Member of The Cato Institute, a privately funded think tank (a body of experts providing ideas and advice on specific economic and political problems). According to their mission statement [22]:

"The mission of the Cato Institute is to originate, disseminate, and increase understanding of public policies based on the principles of individual liberty, limited government, free markets, and peace. Our vision is to create free, open, and civil societies founded on libertarian principles."

Looking over their annual reports (found on their website), I think their mission is straight-forward and their activity fairly transparent, which is why I opt to think that Calabrese's fellowship to Cato does not interfere with his research.

Another contemporary researcher working on hormesis is Suresh Rattan, Ph.D., a biogerontologist (researcher in the field of aging) leading the Laboratory of Cellular Aging at the Department of Molecular Biology and Genetics at the Aarhus University in Denmark.

Since 1976, Dr. Suresh has published more than 230 research and review papers and has authored and edited 14 scientific books and 3 popular science books. As of March 2016, his h-index is 47, which denotes a highly active research career.

I am hopeful to have conveyed the honor and pleasure I feel to present and discuss the work of these illustrious researchers in my attempt to build an argument in support of using positive adaptive stress for better health. Aside of the work of these three researchers, I will also discuss papers written by many other researchers - in a manner as critical as possible (limited to my current knowledge). Before getting into specific topics, I want to provide a modern view of dose response relationships.

Dose Response Relationships

In the fields of toxicology and pharmacology, the dose-response relationship represents a central concept in determining study design, drug manufacturing, and also environmental risk assessment to pollutants.

In The United States, The Environment Protection Agency (EPA) is the organization responsible for developing guidelines and reports regarding dose-response models.

The relationship between dose and response is central to biology because determining the appropriate dose of a certain agent, administered with a certain frequency and for a specific duration can turn that agent from poison to medication.

According to the NIH Office of Science Education (2016) [24], an *"important aspect of dose-response relationships is the concept of threshold"*. They explain it in a very straightforward manner [24]:

"For most types of toxic responses, there is a dose, called a threshold, below which there are no adverse effects from exposure to the chemical. The human body has defenses against many toxic agents. Cells in human organs, especially in the liver and kidneys, break down chemicals into non-toxic substances that can be eliminated from the body in urine and feces."

This is the way in which our bodies can be exposed to toxic insults that are below the threshold and still remain healthy.

The most documented dose-response relationships have been created around a threshold model. In toxicology and in many other fields, a Linear Threshold Model posits that any amount of a toxic agent provided above a certain dose (the threshold) makes it dangerous, while any amount of the same toxic agent provided below the threshold makes it safe. The Linear No Threshold Model (LNT) affirms that any dose, other than zero, of a toxic agent is dangerous (hazardous). The Linear Threshold Model and the Linear No Threshold Model are two opposing concepts. I will provide examples to better understand each.

In radiation, according to the Linear Threshold Model, any amount of radiation below the established threshold is safe, while any amount of radiation above the threshold is dangerous. According to the Linear No Threshold Model, there is no threshold (or the threshold is 0) and any dose, other than 0, is dangerous.

In between these two models, many researchers have proposed the existence of a dose-response relationship (called under different names, sometimes *hormesis*), where low dose exposure, below threshold, to a certain stressor is not only safe (like in the Linear Threshold Model), but it is beneficial and adaptive, while a higher dose (above threshold) exposure would be detrimental. I see this model as being an alteration of the Linear Threshold Model.

Mattson and Calabrese [2] describe it in their effort to define hormesis:

"the response of the cell or organism to the low dose of the toxin that involves an adaptive compensatory process following an initial disruption in homeostasis." [2]

In my understanding, the stressor provokes perturbation in the normal state of the organism (a perturbation of homeostasis - internal equilibrium) that leads to beneficial adaptive mechanisms thereafter.

As an example, think of how weight lifting increases muscle mass: the stressor (the weight) breaks down muscle fibers. As muscle recovers, more fibers are created. Please excuse my gross over-simplification.

Propositions made for this model have been based on hundreds of experiments showing the actual mechanisms. I will describe them later. For now, let us observe a graphic representation of these major models for the sake of better understanding:

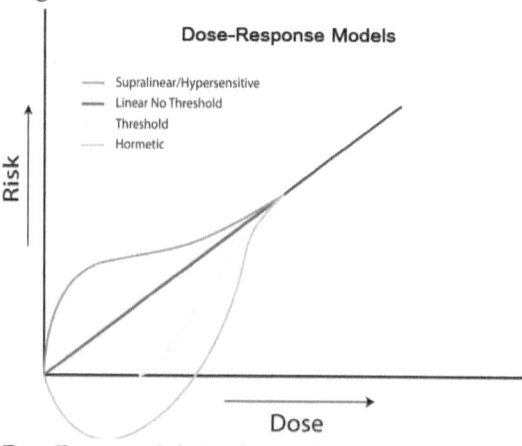

Examples of Dose-Response Relationships. Adapted from Robertson et al. (2013) [25]

Additional to the three models mentioned above, there is a Hypersensitivity Model (blue) that suggests a greater risk at lower doses. The Linear No Threshold (LNT) model (red), as previously described, suggests an increasing risk for doses greater than zero. The Threshold Model (yellow) implies a threshold dose, below which there is no risk and above which the risk increases.

Lastly, the hormesis model proposes for beneficial and adaptive effects at low doses. As one can see from the graphic, hormesis also implies a threshold: low-dose stimulation and high-dose inhibition. This is the biphasic dose response relationship.

Numerous nuclear regulatory agencies and health organizations across the world have adopted the LNT model. Different public and private voices critique this approach as being too conservative and often standing in the way of normal business development.

It is reasonable to think that folks proposing a model different than the LNT are doing so because they would desire more freedom when it comes to the environmental impact of their businesses. A company which, in its normal operations, produces toxic waste, may request eased regulations in terms of their environmental impact because this would allow for running their operations more cheaply.

The Linear No Threshold model (danger at all doses higher than 0) has been initially built based on data from atomic bomb disasters where acute high doses of radiation delivered in a short period of time showed an increased risk of developing cancers. However, since its conception and adoption, there has been research from various fields that does not validate it as a good model.

For example, Cohen (1995) [26] published a study on mortality from lung cancer in which he showed that human response to exposure to low levels of radon is not linear, thus refuting the LNT model.

Another research has found that damage from low level radiation is repaired more efficiently [27]. Similarly, Olipitz et al. (2012) [28] irradiated mice with a dose that was ~400 times higher than natural background radiation for 5 weeks. They did not observe radiation damage, which may indicate that low dose radiation is less damaging, even if the total dose is maintained.

In radiation, the LNT model implies that summing up several small doses will have the same effect as one larger dose; the small doses add up linearly. It also implies that there is no low dose that is considered harmless (safe). Here's another representation of the three most characterized models:

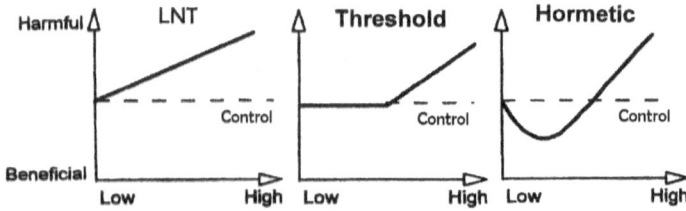

LNT vs. Threshold vs Hormesis. Adapted from Thomas (2013) [145]

Edward Calabrese, one of the leading voices promoting hormesis, published an article in 2011 in the journal *Archives of Toxicology* [29] indicating that Herman J. Muller, creator of the LNT model and Nobel Prize winner in 1946, had access to contradictory evidence but did not disclose it. Some think that:

"Apparently it was a matter of political expediency in an effort to ban above-ground atomic testing." [32]

Calabrese is more critical though, highlighting the implications of not disclosing the information:

"The present assessment of Muller's Nobel Prize Lecture suggests that Muller was deceptive in his presentation, thus profoundly enhancing acceptance of the linear at low-dose modeling and risk assessment practices throughout the second half of the twentieth century to the present." [29]

More recently, organizations like The French Academy of Sciences and The Health Physics Society disproved the LNT model - at least in the context of radiation. The French Academy of Sciences supports hormesis [30], while The Health Physics Society rejects the LNT model providing different arguments for their rationale [31].

Similarly, an in-depth review published in *RSNA Radiology* in 2009 noted that LNT is inconsistent with radiation biology and experimental data [34]:

"Biologic data demonstrate that the defense mechanisms against radiation-induced carcinogenesis are powerful and diverse. This is not surprising, because organisms have been subjected to reactive oxygen species from physiologic processes and environmental insults during evolution.

Life is characterized by the ability to build defenses against toxic agents, whether internal or environmental. The defenses are overwhelmed at high doses and are stimulated at low doses, which is incompatible with the LNT model." [34]

In their conclusion, they say that LNT was a useful model in the past (half a century ago) and that current regulations on radiation protection should be based on concepts and facts that are drawn from current scientific data, and not from opinion. Moreover, they say that [34]:

"Preconceived concepts impede progress; in the case of the LNT model, they have resulted in substantial medical, economic, and other societal harm."

In my view, regulators are doing a good job when trying to protect the public from the dangers of different toxic compounds.

I also think that LNT may have to be approached contextually. This model, even though widely accepted and implemented by regulators, has been the subject of many controversies and attacks; and many of these attacks and contradictory arguments may be legitimate. However, regulators and policy makers still adhere to it because it is conservative. They think that other models may be underestimating risks.

To a certain extent, LNT may seem a good model in terms of protection from ionizing radiation. But, are there ways to make it better?

Regulators could investigate what these opposing voices say about hormesis and ionizing radiation. This way, it would become clearer if these opposing voices are indeed only trying to protect whatever financial interest they may have or if their arguments are solid from a scientific perspective.

Understanding Hormesis

These dose-response models, threshold and no-threshold, receive a lot of attention and are highly debatable in the context of radiation. There may be different interests at stake (financial and non-financial). My purpose with this book is not to discuss these models, but to distinguish them and make a point that different levels of a stressor can be beneficial or detrimental. Whether this is reflective of mechanisms that could be put under the *hormesis* umbrella is not important to me. I am using the word *hormesis* several times throughout the book merely because of its clear description by its most avid proponents.

Zooming out of radiation biology, here is Mattson and Calabrese's graphical representation of hormesis [2]:

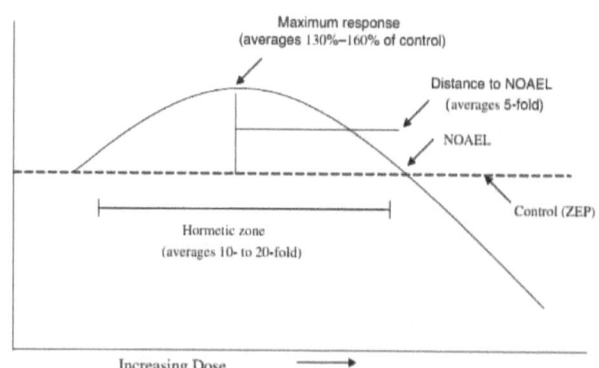

Fig. 1 Dose-response curve showing the quantitative features of hormesis. NOAEL, no observed adverse effect level; ZEP, zero equivalent point (ZEP) (i.e., value equal to the control value)

Adapted from Mattson and Calabrese (2009) [2]

This model, built on numerous observed dose-response effects (from drugs, food compounds, toxic chemicals, etc.), is somewhat incomprehensible compared to previous representations from this book. What I am getting as the important message from this graphic is that the maximum stimulatory (positive) response from a certain dose of a stressor is within the range of 30% to 60% greater doses, compared to control values.

This would be, by Mattson and Calabrese's standards, the sweet spot dose (130% to 160%) - the dose of a stressor at which one can derive the maximum benefits. How this may change through time, with habituation and tolerance, remains discussable.

Here is another, more straightforward, illustration that may make you better understand this dose-response relationship model [33]:

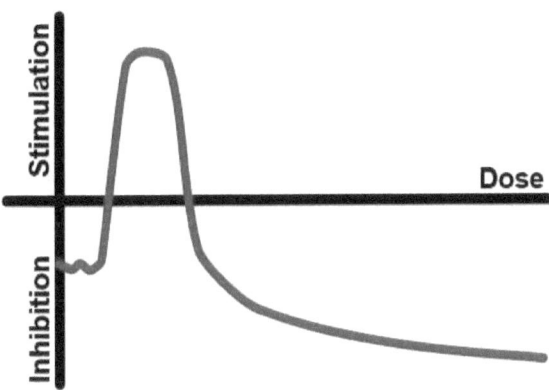

Hormesis - Dose-Response Curve. Adapted from [33]

One of the reasons that I refrain from embracing the conceptualization of this mechanism using the word *hormesis* is that the term has not been widely accepted within the scientific community and also because it may produce controversies in the field of radiation and not only. Most importantly, I do not need to use *hormesis* to describe a biphasic dose response relationship.

Plus, this biphasic dose response mechanism, low-dose stimulation high-dose inhibition, has been described with different terms since the beginning of the modern scientific literature. Some of them are [2]:

- U-shaped,
- inverted U-shaped,
- bidirectional,
- J-shaped,
- biphasic,
- dual effects,
- Arndt-Schulz law,
- hormesis,
- bimodal,
- bell-shaped curve,
- paradoxical effects,
- pharmacological inversion,
- functional antagonism,
- and several other names.

All of these terms describe the same mechanism. Together, they have gathered a couple of thousands of citations in the scientific literature, beginning in 1945 and until 2007 [2].

I used Google Scholar in March 2016 to search for 'hormesis'. I filtered the results and limited the search for the years 2007 - 2016. My search returned 14,400 results. I made the same search on Pubmed and I got ~880 results. So, this term, hormesis, seems to be receiving much more traction than it has in all its history combined.

A widely cited review from 2012 was published in *Endocrine Reviews*. The purpose was to explore low-dose effects and non-monotonic dose-responses (different from LNT) of hormone and endocrine disrupting chemicals. The review did not seek to prove or validate hormesis, but to show that biologically toxic chemicals can have different and non-monotonic (non-linear) effects at different doses [35].

Examples of Biphasic Dose Response Relationships

To provide evidence for the biphasic dose-response relationship, Mattson and Calabrese [2] have built a large database of ~8,000 observed effects. Some of these effects are seen in or with respect to:

- neuroscience data
- anxiolytic drugs
- antiseizure drugs
- pain and stress responses
- environmental contaminants
- hormones and neurotransmitters
- low-dose stimulation of tumors
- low-dose stimulation of microbes by antibiotics
- osteoporosis
- and many other areas.

The impact of these effects on biology is well described by Mattson and Calabrese, who provide specific examples [2]. Here are a few:

Aging - low-dose stress increases longevity
Bone - low-dose bisphosphonates strengthen bones
Cancer - low-dose usage of numerous anti-tumor drugs increase the growth of tumor cells
Cardiovascular Disease - low-dose statins act on vasculature
HIV - low-dose antiviral drugs increase virus proliferation
Antibiotics - low-dose antibiotics may lead to bacterial growth

Nutrition - low-doses of phytochemicals in food and metals in water may have adaptive positive effects on health

Nutrition - food deprivation and fasting can increase resilience

Alcohol - low-dose intake considered beneficial in certain circumstances (although its effects have been exaggerated, in my view)

Exercise - short-burst intense exercise (fighting, sprinting, etc) may be more beneficial than steady-state prolonged exercise (mitochondrial hormesis).

In terms of drugs [2]:

Aspirin:

- protects from myocardial infarction at low-doses
- can reduce pain at higher doses, but it can also increase the risk of developing ulcers

Diazepam (Valium):

- reduces anxiety at low-doses
- alters cognition and motor function at higher doses

Antidepressants (Prozac and Paxil):

- stimulate BDNF (brain derived neurotrophic factor) at low-doses
- can have detrimental effects at higher doses

Metformin:

"The widely prescribed diabetes drug metformin may act, in part, by inducing a mild stress in the muscle cells similar to what occurs during exercise. Both exercise and metformin stimulate the activity of a protein called AMP-activated protein kinase (AMPK), resulting in increased sensitivity of muscle cells to insulin." [2]

To note is that for some of the actions of these chemicals there is no clear *hormesis*-like mechanism, the observed mechanism being more dependent on threshold. Similarly, Mattson and Calabrese [2] do not explain or provide reference for the negative effects when some of these compounds are given at high doses. I think it would be inappropriate to generalize or to try to find a dose-response relationship that would fit all scenarios.

We have seen that some processes are better described by linear no threshold curves, others by threshold curves, others by hormesis-like curves. Assigning an appropriate curve to each observable phenomenon is more desirable than trying to fit all phenomena under a single dose-response curve. This is one of the reasons why I provided a few examples from different aspects of life, where dual dose-response relationships may be more appropriate.

The authors [2] report biphasic responses for chemical agents like arsenic, mercury, radiation, pesticides and a host of other agents in organisms ranging from yeasts, worms, flies, mice, humans and many others. In terms of human health, they become more specific on the biphasic effects of some minerals and vitamins:

Selenium:

- critical for health (supports the functions of more than 30 selenoproteins)
- sufficient at low doses, toxic and life-threatening at high-doses

In an article published in *Scientific American* in 2015, Mark Mattson exemplified [36]:

"Eating too many Brazil nuts can poison the liver and lungs because of the presence of the trace element selenium. Yet eating just a few supplies

an essential nutrient that is incorporated into an enzyme that may help protect against heart disease and cancer."

Vitamin D:

- critical for bone health and wound healing
- sufficient at low to moderate doses, toxic at high doses

A similar trend has been observed when measuring blood levels of vitamin D (25OHD) [37]:

- deficiency at < 20ng/mL
- insufficiency at levels 20 - 40 ng/mL
- proposed optimal at levels 40 - 60 ng/mL
- toxicity at levels > 80 ng/mL

Vitamin A:

- required for the development of multiple organs, critical for eye health
- in excess, it can lead to liver damage and osteoporosis

Iron:

"Iron is essential for red blood cell health and also serves important regulatory functions in other cell types, but excessive iron intake can cause oxidative damage to tissues." [2]

Adaptive Cellular Stress Responses

Reactive Oxygen Species:

- cellular low-dose free radicals promote the activation of ACSRPs (adaptive cell stress response pathways)
- cellular high-dose free radicals can be damaging

Superoxide (free radical) is converted to hydrogen peroxide and oxygen by the enzyme superoxide dismutase (SOD). Hydrogen peroxide is then partially reduced to hydroxyl radical or fully reduced to water by the action of enzymes like catalase and glutathione peroxidase.

"Thus, levels of superoxide are normally kept low. However, high amounts of superoxide can occur in certain conditions (e.g., with reductions in levels of antioxidant enzymes) and can damage cells by conversion to more highly reactive free radicals, including hydroxyl radical and (by interaction with nitric oxide)." [2]

Similarly, Mattson and Calabrese [2] hypothesize that the adaptive response to low levels of stressors allowed organisms to expand the range of environments in which they can survive. The first example that comes to my mind is human skin pigmentation in different climates (darker in warmer climates, lighter in colder climates).

Adaptive cellular stress response pathways (ACSRPs) are metabolic pathways that respond to oxidative stress by promoting cellular repair and survival [38]. Some of these include, but are not limited to: the Nrf2-ARE pathway, the NF-κB pathway, and the sirtuin-FOXO pathway. Signals that modulate these pathways include: exercise, drugs, dietary restriction, cognitive stimulation (mild psychologic stress), and phytochemicals [38].

Specific examples of phytochemicals [2]:

- sulphoraphane (in broccoli) can modulate Nrf2 and Keap1
- curcumin interacts with Nrf2
- resveratrol (in red grapes) activates sirtuins
- allicin (in garlic) can promote calcium influx by activating membrane TRP channels.

"When exposed to plant chemicals such as curcumin or the sulforaphane in broccoli, Keap1 releases Nrf2, which then moves into the cell nucleus. There it activates genes that encode antioxidant enzymes that eliminate free radicals. Sulforaphane stimulates the Nrf2 pathway to rid the body of an overabundance of free radicals." [36]

More details about how these pathways and cellular mechanisms are activated will be provided later in the book.

Dose and Context are very Important

As we have seen, stressors administered at varying doses lead to different responses. Important consideration and assessment need to be provided also to: the duration and frequency of exposure, the constancy of the dosage (increasing, constant, decreasing), as well as the context in which the stressor is being provided.

For example, we've learned about the importance of antioxidants (vitamins A, C, and E) on human health. The general public may be confused though. You often hear in the news how supplementing with a certain vitamin and/or antioxidant can not only have neutral effects, but it can even be detrimental. Why is that?

One possible argument is that the metabolic picture is much different when using a vitamin in isolation (by supplementing with it) compared to consuming a plant food that is rich in that vitamin. The plant food may also contain other factors that allow the vitamin to be processed in a beneficial way. Mattson [36] explains:

"Bitter-tasting chemicals made by plants act as natural pesticides. When we eat plant-based foods, we consume low levels of these toxic chemicals, which mildly stresses cells in the body in much the same way that exercise or going without food for long periods does. The cells do not

die—in fact, they get stronger because their response to the stress shores up their ability to adapt to still more stress."

Moreover [36]:

"Dousing the body with supplements may inhibit the natural stress response throughout the body. In one 2009 study researchers at Friedrich Schiller University Jena in Germany and their colleagues showed that after a month of exercising and taking antioxidant supplements, a group of men had no improvement in regulation of blood glucose and other health indicators, whereas men who only exercised did benefit."

Mattson [36] thinks that supplementing with the antioxidant may have negated the positive adaptive effects of the exercise alone. Therefore [2]:

"Not only is the dose a critical determinant of whether an environmental challenge is beneficial or damaging, but in addition the frequency of exposure is key because cells must have time to recover to benefit from the stress. The importance of a recovery period for the accrual of the benefits of exercise is widely recognized."

Here we are reminded of the clear distinction between hormesis (a biphasic dose-response relationship) and homeopathy [36]:

"...hormesis works and differentiates it from homeopathy, which claims, without valid evidence or a plausible mechanism, that vanishingly small amounts of what causes illness can be curative."

While Mattson makes this distinction in a reputable journal [36], Calabrese published an article about hormesis in a homeopathy journal. Even though most of Calabrese's work, that I have read, shows good research conduit, this action may not serve to promote the clean (scientific and evidence based) name of hormesis that he wishes to promote [39].

Mattson and Calabrese think that one of the major goals of medicine and pharmacology should be to decide upon the dose and the frequency of administration of a certain compound so that relief of symptoms is maximized, while side effects are minimized [2].

The most common approach for treatment with drugs and supplements is to use a constant or an increasing dose. In many circumstances, the individual builds tolerance for the dose at hand, and increasing the dose may increase the risk for toxicity. Hence, a recovery (deprivation) period would serve as sensitizing the individual to the certain chemical.

As you may see, this is a rather complex approach and many people may refrain from using it, thus potentially negating the positive effects from a certain drug, supplement, compound, or stressor.

As previously mentioned, my focus is to discuss stress physiology and not to prove hormesis. I want to acknowledge the existence of physiologically different responses to stressors that are administered at varying levels, thus promoting the existence of different dose-response relationships.

Up to this point I have told you that:

- some stressors can be detrimental at any dose greater than zero (Linear No Threshold Model)
- some stressors may have no effect at low-level doses, while being toxic after a certain level (Threshold Model)
- some stressors may provide beneficial adaptive responses at low levels and until a certain threshold is met, while they may become

toxic above the threshold (biphasic dose response model - often mentioned as hormesis)

- some stressors may show markedly increased toxicity at lower levels and a slowly increasing toxicity below the threshold (Supralinear Model)

While these are the most encountered dose-response relationship models for stressors, there certainly exist more. Promoting a generalizable model to be applied in all circumstances may, thus, be non-sensical.

Throughout this book, one of my purposes is to exemplify with research studies and my personal (anecdotal) experience about how we could make use of stressors (exercise, phytochemicals, fasting, drugs, toxins, cognitive challenges, toxins, etc) to increase tolerance, resilience and to induce positive physiologic and psychologic adaptations.

I will begin the following chapter with an in-depth insight into the biology of stress.

Stress and Adaptation in Physiology

Chapter 2:
Stressors and Adaptive Responses

Less work to get more time for what? More pay to do what? Few people give much thought to what they will do with their free time and extra money after they have reached a comfortable minimum income.

Hans Selye

Biological systems gravitate toward homeostasis, or the maintenance of a state of internal constancy. Challenges, stressors, and other disrupting factors may push homeostasis to a new, more resilient level if their action on the system is not too overwhelming, destructive, or lethal.

Here I am going to examine some of the mechanisms of biologic stressors, aiming to derive insights that could improve human life. I will start with a historical view of physiologic stress by introducing the extensive work of Hans Selye, a pioneering endocrinologist of the 20th century.

Stress - The Beginnings

Hans Selye (1907 - 1982) of Austro-Hungarian origins has often been considered the Einstein of medical research, mostly *"because of his reliance and emphasis on creativity and originality in medical research"* [42]. Szabo et al. (2012) consider him an 'outlier' by modern definition due to his extreme productivity [42]. During his 30-year period of active scientific career, Selye published more than 1,500 articles, authored more than 30 books and often worked 12 hours a day, 7 days a week. As other researchers who worked for him recall: *"it is not surprising that he discovered more than the stress syndrome"* [42].

Even though he coined the term 'biologic stress response', Selye was not the first to use the word 'stress'. He described mechanisms of stress response in a widely cited letter to the editor of *Nature* sent on May 18, 1936 [43]:

"Experiments on rats show that if the organism is severely damaged by acute non-specific nocuous agents such as exposure to cold, surgical injury, production of spinal shock (transcision of the cord), excessive muscular exercise, or intoxications with sub-lethal doses of diverse drugs (adrenaline, atropine, morphine, formaldehyde, etc.), a typical syndrome appears, the symptoms of which are independent of the nature of the damaging agent or the pharmacological type of the drug employed, and represent rather a response to damage as such." [43]

He later named this response as *The General Adaptation Syndrome* (G.A.S.) and he described it as consisting of three phases: the alarm reaction, the stage of resistance, and the stage of exhaustion [44].

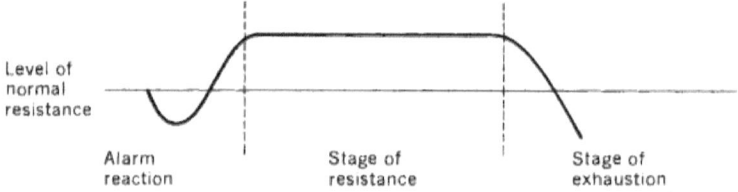

Stages of the General Adaptation Syndrome. Adapted from [44]

The first time Selye suspected the existence of the G.A.S. was in 1925 while studying medicine at the University of Prague:

"During one of the initial lectures in internal medicine, we were shown several patients in the earliest stages of various infectious diseases. The professor carefully pointed out all the specific signs and symptoms characteristic of each disease but what struck me most was that each of these patients felt and looked ill, had a coated tongue, and complained of more or less diffuse aches and pains in the joints and of intestinal disturbances with loss of appetite and loss of weight." [44]

Selye noted a *common syndrome* in these patients (G.A.S.), a syndrome characterized by nonspecific signs which passed as unimportant to the physician, as they would not help in accurately making a diagnosis for their illnesses [44]:

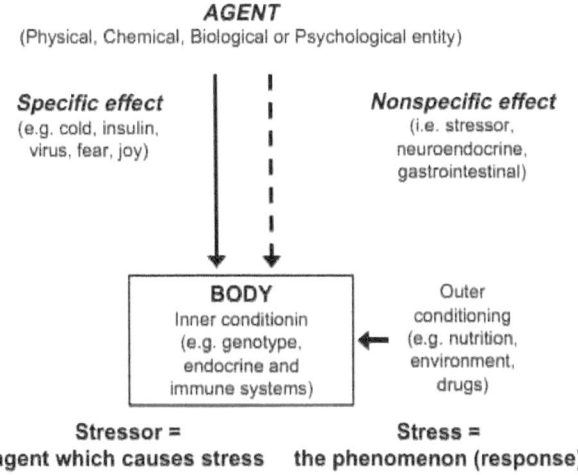

AGENT
(Physical, Chemical, Biological or Psychological entity)

Specific effect
(e.g. cold, insulin, virus, fear, joy)

Nonspecific effect
(i.e. stressor, neuroendocrine, gastrointestinal)

BODY
Inner conditionin
(e.g. genotype, endocrine and immune systems)

Outer conditioning
(e.g. nutrition, environment, drugs)

Stressor =
agent which causes stress

Stress =
the phenomenon (response)

Specific and Nonspecific Effects. Adapted from [42]

During the first stage of G.A.S., an organism shows a response characteristic of the first exposure to a stressor. At the same time, according to Selye (2013), *"its resistance is diminished and, if the stressor is sufficiently strong (severe burns, extremes of temperature), death may result"* [44].

While deliberate exposure to cold temperature may elicit health benefits, it may not be wise for a *newbie* to jump into an ice bath and stay there for 30 minutes. The acute dose of the stressor (cold) may be too high; chances are that negative outcomes will follow. Starting with a small dose and progressively increasing it over time may be a better strategy, should one decide to use cold exposure to gain some health benefits.

In the second stage of the G.A.S., Selye (2013) explains that if continued exposure to the stressor is compatible with adaptation (that is: if the stressor is not too overwhelming to kill the organism), the stage of resistance follows. In this phase, the signs of the alarm reaction have disappeared and resistance goes above normal levels.

Selye hypothesized that the increased resistance to the persisting stressor is finite (adaptation energy). Hence, the stage of resistance terminates when this adaptation energy is depleted. At this point, *"the signs of the alarm reaction reappear, but now they are irreversible, and the individual dies"* [44]. Let me try to put G.A.S. in the context of cold exposure:

1. A healthy person takes a cold bath for the first time for 5 minutes (no ice). The stress is not lethal. An adaptive response may occur.

2. The second stage of resistance ensues when no signs of the alarm reaction are present. Increasing the dose by increasing the exposure time or by decreasing water temperature or both could possibly result in health benefits. Thus, to elicit such benefits, I assume it requires remaining within the first two stages.

3. If the initial stressor persists for too long or if subsequent higher doses of the stressor are received chronically, negative consequences may follow.

Selye often saw the three stages of G.A.S. as being analogous to human life [44]:

Childhood - low resistance, excessive responses to stimuli
Adulthood - adaptation to the most common agents has occurred => higher resistance
Old age - irreversible loss of adaptability => exhaustion, death.

With his multi-decade research career, Hans Selye laid the groundwork for stress physiology. In my opinion, he should represent a role model of productivity and creativity for aspiring researchers; he represents one for me.

As time passed and as others built on top of his research, more terms describing the mechanisms of stress have emerged. Most of them relate to the same phenomena, while some of them deviate (more or less) from the physiology of stress.

Biological Stress Response Terminology

The current disparity in terminology with regards to biological stress response may have risen from a lack of frequent interaction among scientists and researchers in many areas. Thus, dose-response relationships have been described in the literature using a multitude of terms.

A paper from 2007, which has 58 authors, mentions some of the terms used to describe the shape of the dose-response relationship curve seen in many systems subjected to stress [45]:

- β-curve
- biphasic
- bell-shaped
- U-shaped
- inverted-U shaped
- J-shaped
- diphasic
- bitonic
- bimodal
- bidirectional
- sinusoidal
- subsidy gradient
- functional antagonism
- dual response

- nonmonotonic
- stimulatory-inhibitory
- and others.

Similarly, *"terms such as autoprotection, heteroprotection, adaptive response, preconditioning, hormesis, xenohormesis, paradoxical and others have characterized the shape of the dose-response patterns mentioned above when low doses elicit an adaptive response of the cell/organism."* [45]

The mechanism that is common in adaptive response, conditioning, and autoprotection is that exposure to low level stressors activates molecular pathways that increase an organism's ability to withstand subsequent, more severe levels of stressors.

As Calabrese et al. (2007) [45] pointed out, biological systems do not 'care' about the exact terminology used to describe their response to stress and stressors:

"When biological systems are exposed to a low dose of a toxicant or other mild stress, survival will typically be enhanced when physiologically existing mechanisms that protect against a similar but more severe stress are activated or upregulated." [45]

Stressors, Stress, and Resilience

The concept of resilience will often be encountered and described throughout this book. Resilience has mostly been discussed in psychology related contexts; thus, I consider it is important to define it from a biologic perspective.

Most simplistically put, (biologic) resilience is the ability of a system to cope with stressors. It is the ability to respond to perturbations by resisting damage and by quick recovery. Stressors can come in many forms [46]:

- perturbations of/from the external environment - heat, cold, etc.
- perturbations of/from the internal environment (endogenous) - high blood glucose, infections, psychologic stressors, etc.

The dose and the duration of exposure are important in determining the likelihood for positive adaptation to occur and for shifting the system (organism) into a higher utility basin: too big of a dose of a stressor delivered acutely could lead to death, while too small of a dose may not trigger any adaptive mechanism. Oken and colleagues (2015) [46] exemplify:

"In an athletics example, both short-term stress at an Olympic competition and longer-term stress from high effort athletic activity over a training period may improve athletic performance. However, excessive or repeated perturbations may have a cost to the underlying system that outweighs the benefit." [46]

Physiologic stress responses leading to adaptive mechanisms include, but are not limited to [46]:

- activation of the HPA axis (hypothalamus-pituitary-adrenal axis)
- activation of the norepinephrine-sympathetic nervous system
- activation of the parasympathetic nervous system
- expression/silencing of certain genes
- modulation of the immune system
- etc.

Oken et al. (2015) think that restricting the immune system from being exposed to sufficient foreign substances could result in over-reactivity to such substances and the development of allergies [46]. This is in agreement with the theory that farm-raised children could be healthier than those raised in urban areas because of their increased exposure to a variety of environmental agents; their immune systems are more challenged/trained.

Stress and Adaptation in Physiology

Physiologic stress responses can usually be measured or quantified through markers such as: blood pressure, heart rate, catecholamine release, and electro-dermal activity, to name just a few [46].

Stressors affect homeostasis. Perturbing factors induce stress responses, thereby increasing tolerance and activating coping mechanisms. Better tolerance promotes a higher utility function. It moves homeostasis to an upgraded level. The multitude of such processes can be explored under the umbrella of adaptive homeostasis.

Adaptive Homeostasis

Davies (2016) [47] describes adaptive homeostasis as being the contraction or expansion of the homeostatic range in response to different perturbing agents. Davies considers that the contraction of the homeostatic range occurs when perturbing agents are removed, while expansion occurs when an organism is exposed to sub-toxic and non-damaging agents.

I think Davies is conservative when describing the expansion of the homeostatic range/limit. I am inclined to say that it occurs when an organism is exposed to a perturbing or damaging, but non-lethal, agent.

Homeostasis, as seen in Guyton's *Textbook of Medical Physiology* (1991) [47, 48]:

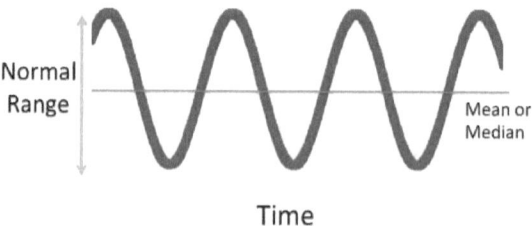

Homeostasis. Adapted from [47]

Homeostasis is a characteristic of numerous biologic and physiologic functions, including: heart rate, blood pressure, blood glucose levels, the ratio of NAD+ to NADH, core temperature, etc [47].

Others have proposed theories to expand the homeostasis model by including terms such as allostasis, allostatic load, and heterostasis. In short [49]:

Homeostasis - focus on steady state (equilibrium) and optimal set points
Allostasis - focus on optimal operating ranges
Allostatic load - long-term cost of allostasis; reflects the accumulated damage of prolonged action of stressors.

One of the major differences between the homeostasis model and the allostasis model is that allostasis may lead to pathology. Schulkin (2004) [50] explains it better:

Homeostasis	Allostasis
Normal setpoint	Changing setpoint
Physiologic equilibrium	Compensated equilibrium
No anticipation of demand	Anticipation of demand
No adjustment based on history	Adjustment based on history
Adjustment carries no price	Adjustment and accomodation carry a price
No pathology	Leads to pathology

Homeostasis vs. Allostasis. Adapted from [50]

Exploring the similarities and differences between these concepts is not part of the agenda of this book. Next, I will elaborate on the mechanisms of adaptive homeostasis and how to expand the range within which biologic systems can function properly.

Davies (2016) proposes the use of 'adaptive homeostasis' to describe stress response. He thinks that terms such as hormesis, allostasis and heterostasis are inaccurate descriptors of molecular and cellular stress responses. In one of his recent papers, he offered a graphical depiction of the concept [47]:

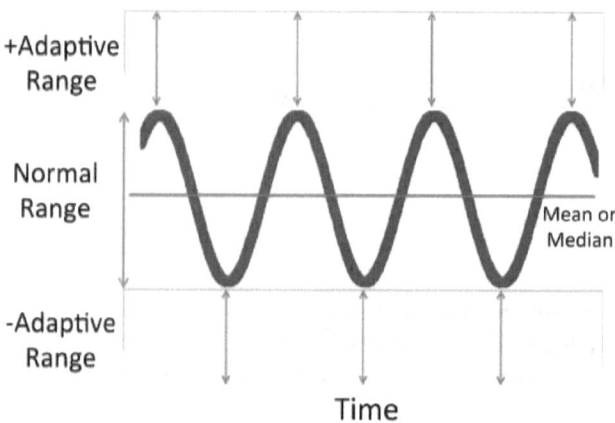

Adaptive Homeostasis - proposed by Davies (2016). Adapted from [47]

In addition to the homeostatic range (normal), positive and negative adaptive ranges can be induced as a response to the action of stressors. He provides examples for both.

Positive adaptive homeostasis occurs, for example, when a signal given by nanomolar levels of hydrogen peroxide (an R.O.S. - reactive oxygen species) increases the synthesis of proteasome (protein complex that degrades damaged proteins), immunoproteasome, and other similar cellular regulators for up to several hours. This happens via the Nrf2-Keap1 pathway. Davies (2016) explains:

"In response to a wide variety of electrophiles and oxidants, Nrf2 avoids proteolytic digestion, undergoes phosphorylation, and translocates to the nucleus where it binds to Electrophile Response Elements (EPREs) which are also called Antioxidant Response Elements (AREs) within target gene sequences." [47]

When Nrf2 binds to a gene's ARE/EPRE, it increases the expression of that gene and this leads to a transient increase in the homeostatic range.

Negative adaptive homeostasis occurs (for that same example) with the loss of the signal given by hydrogen peroxide. This allows the system to return within its homeostatic range.

Another example of negative adaptive homeostasis, provided by Davies (2016), occurs when an organism consumes a lot of protein:

"Similarly, when organisms are exposed to a diet rich in amino acids, they turn off production of amino acid synthetases, thus decreasing capacity to synthesize amino acids. Restoration of a 'normal' diet would then reverse the transient decrease in capacity back within the normal homeostatic range." [47]

Even though these concepts may now seem abstract and hard to grasp, my purpose is to expand on them using relevant examples in the remaining pages of the book. Moreover, I bring them to attention because they have been described (with different terminology) in the scientific literature and they are currently tested and researched by scientists such as Kelvin Davies of U.S.C, Mark P. Mattson of the N.I.A., John C. Wingfield of U.S.C., Michael Ristow of E.T.H. Zurich, and others who I will further familiarize you with.

Timing and Duration

The capacity to adapt and cope with higher levels of a physiologic or psychologic stressor is dependent on the intensity and duration of the previous exposure to that stressor. Let me exemplify this within the context of cold temperature stress.

As I mentioned earlier, it may not be wise for your first exposure to cold stress to jump straight into an ice cold river and remain in the water for 20 minutes; chances are that you may develop hypothermia. A better alternative may be to start at home in the safety of your bathroom, with mixed/alternating showers (warm + cold water, intermittently for a couple of minutes) or by taking brief cold showers. As you develop tolerance to a certain dose of cold, as you adapt (habituate) to it, you could increase the time you remain under the cold shower (thus, modifying the dose). Then, you could gradually shift to taking cold baths, and eventually ice baths.

When you get used to a certain dose of a certain stressor, when you develop tolerance, the curve of positive adaptation flattens out. To keep leveraging the positive adaptive effects, you may have to titrate the dose, frequency, and/or duration of exposure to the stressor.

In this case, when you 'graduate' to taking ice-baths, the next iteration would be to increase the duration of exposure. When you reach the level of getting perturbed only by very long-ice baths (that is, when you become very tolerant, resistant, and adapted to cold), one possible, subsequent strategy would be the use of a re-sensitization period.

Withdrawing from cold exposure for a while (weeks to months) may reset your tolerance and you could start the entire process all over again, with a lower dose, frequency and duration of exposure. This way, you could engage in a never ending cycle of exposure, constantly reaping the possible, somewhat controversial and debatable, benefits of this practice.

I exemplified using cold exposure because I think that it makes for a pertinent explanation of conditioning, tolerance buildup, and adaptation to perturbing agents. Nonetheless, you could replace cold stress with any other stressor or perturbing agent, including but not limited to: heat stress, fasting, intermittent fasting, ketosis, caloric restriction, hypergravity, supplementation, use of pharmaceuticals, plant phytochemicals, allergens, environmental toxins, deliberate cognitive stress, etc.

Maintaining an increased sensitivity to a stressor with the purpose of continuously reaping potential benefits is the result of constantly changing/altering the strategy: increasing/decreasing the dose, frequency and the duration of exposure. The concepts of pre- and post-conditioning are worth mentioning here.

In their book about hormesis, Suresh and Le Bourg (2014) [51] claim that pre-conditioning is known by a multitude of terms, such as: tolerance, adaptive response, desensitization, and reprogramming:

"Both in pre- and in postconditioning, it has been observed that there is a limited time frame in which the low-dose application (mild stressor condition) can exert a beneficial effect. Biological systems will react to mild stress conditions if they are in a state of (enhanced) sensitivity." [51]

Preconditioning simply means: exposure to a stressor in order to be (better) prepared for future encounters with that stressor.

In vaccination, one is exposed to a weak version of a virus to train the immune system to recognize and be able to efficiently deal with future encounters with the live virus. Postconditioning refers to an exposure to a milder version of a stressor, after an initial acute and more intense dose of that stressor.

Post-conditioning is most often discussed in the context of myocardial infarction and it is *"achieved by repetitive occlusion and reperfusion in the early minutes after revascularization of acute myocardial infarction"* [52]. Both pre- and post-conditioning are known as powerful tools to provide protection against myocardial ischemia (when the heart tissue is deprived of oxygen and nutrients; ischemia can lead to heart attack).

Suresh and Le Bourg (2014) explain pre- and post-conditioning with an example of survival rates in cells exposed to heat stress compared to normal cells [51]:

1. Cells are exposed to heat, then are incubated at normal temperature
2. Cells are exposed to heat again - to determine if they developed tolerance

"Preconditioned cells survive this high temperature in comparison with non-pretreated cells. Examination of the kinetics of induction and decay of thermotolerance showed that an interval of about 4–8 hours at normal temperature was required before the maximum thermotolerance manifested itself." [51]

In post-conditioning, they recommend allowing *"not too short nor too long"* time between the administration of a severe dose of stress and the administration of a milder dose of stress [51].

In my translation, to maintain sensitivity, exposure to a high-dose of heat stress should be followed (not immediately) by exposure to a milder dose of heat stress. Suresh and Le Bourg (2014) explain that the enhanced sensitivity following a severe stress exposure depends on the time and the temperature of the initial heat treatment [51].

Benefits from stressors timed and dosed appropriately are obtained, most likely, because of the adaptive, recuperative mechanisms that follow. Such mechanisms increase resilience. Stressors timed and dosed inappropriately may be without effect or detrimental. In the context of cold exposure, it may be ineffective to take cold showers when one is adapted to taking prolonged ice baths.

I will briefly mention the concept of cross-tolerance, or how exposure and adaptation to a certain stressor can provide adaptation to different stressors.

Suresh and Le Bourg (2014) exemplify how adaptation to heat stress can provide resistance to oxidant stress [51]. I will return to this, in more detail, later in the book.

In their discussion of physiologic stress, Suresh and Le Bourg (2014) adopt the use of 'hormesis', motivating that its key features imply the disruption of homeostasis, *"activation of corrective cellular pathways that lead to modest overcompensation, the reestablishment of homeostasis, and the adaptive nature of the process on future exposure to stressors."* [51]

Instead of adding terminology that could complicate the understanding of physiologic stress and adaptive responses, I would personally focus on eliminating or keeping the current terminology, unless it is extremely necessary and it would provide tremendous benefits, which I do not see the case for here (for hormesis). This is why I am not in favor of the use of 'hormesis', despite the fact that much of the recent research literature on physiologic stress is tagged with this word. Putting this aside, let me, next, discuss cellular and molecular stress responses.

Molecular Stress Response

Up to 5% of the genomes of most uni- and multi-cellular species codes for GPCR, the heptahelical G protein-coupled receptor that allows organisms to sense their environment. According to Chadwick and Maudsley (2010):

Stress and Adaptation in Physiology

"The GPCR system has adapted to perceive almost all forms of environmental entities, for example, photons, odorants, lipids, carbohydrates, peptides, and nucleic acids. The GPCR system has also likely adapted to the presence of exogenous compounds that may at some doses be deleterious but at lower levels may indeed possess beneficial actions." [136]

The plasticity of a GPCR system may provide an organism the maintenance of beneficial sensitivity, so that it could be able to cope with future changes within its environment. It should, therefore, not come as a surprise that certain living beings may have been adapted to use the environment with its agents (either beneficial or poisonous) in support of their biochemical status:

"Such an advantage may have secured the capacity of early life forms to take a foothold in the harsh primordial terrestrial or oceanic environments." [136]

Some of such agents elicit stress upon the organism, regardless of their poisonous/non-poisonous nature. To survive, the organism responds adaptively. Some researchers highlight three major aspects of this stress response [53]:

1. Immediate SR
2. Delayed SR
3. Downstream Effects

The immediate stress response involves receptors and cell signals and their activity upon the exposure to the stressor, while the delayed stress response involves the activity of receptors and cell signals in the presence or after the removal of the stressor. The third major aspect of stress response deals with downstream mechanisms to counteract the effects of the stressor with the purpose of reestablishing homeodynamics.

Taken at different levels (cell, organ, organism), stress response manifestations include: apoptosis (programmed cell death), inflammation, thermoregulation, as well as hyper-adrenocorticism (often known as Cushing's Syndrome). Demirovic et al. (2014) discuss about a few stressor and the responses they trigger [53]:

Response Name	Stressors
HSR	Heat, heavy metals, antibiotics, denatured proteins
OSR	Free radicals, ROS, pro-oxidants, low levels of oxygen
NSR	Food limitation, hypoxia, damaged organelles
ESR or sirtuin response	Energy depletion
DDR	Radiation, oxidants, free radicals, ROS
UPR or ER stress response	Unfolded and misfolded proteins in ER
ISR	Pathogens, allergens, damaged macromolecules

Demirovic et al. (2014) [53] - Excerpt adapted from Table 12.1

The heat shock response (HSR) is triggered by various stressors (as seen above) and it involves the synthesis of heat shock proteins (HSP; often known as stress proteins) that act in protein remodeling, protein refolding, prevention of protein aggregation, and stimulation of proteolysis (protein degradation). HSPs are considered essential for survival in case of severe stress [53]. Two of their primary purposes include the maintenance of protein structure and integrity.

Demirovic and colleagues (2014) report several studies conducted in yeasts, worms, flies, rodents, and human cells which have mentioned health promoting effects of stressors that act via the HSR system [53]. They called them *HSR-inducing hormetins*. The nomenclature is probably derived from the concept of hormesis; you may see why I think of this as being an unnecessary complication.

"Such HSR-mediating hormetins include physical exercise, thermal stress, and some plant extracts, for example, the Chinese herb Sanchi. Although some questions have been raised about the wider application of heat as a hormetin, thermal hormesis for humans through HSR induction is also being reported." [53]

The **oxidative stress response** (OSR) is how cells defend against oxidative stress. The response is mediated by Nrf2, a nuclear factor which controls the expression of numerous genes whose proteins are involved in detoxifying and eliminating oxidants and electrophilic agents, thus increasing the antioxidant potential of the cell [53]:

"Nrf2 is ubiquitously expressed in all tissues, with the highest concentrations in the kidney, muscle, lung, heart, liver, and brain." [53]

Factors known to activate OSR include reactive oxygen species, hypoxia, pro-oxidant plant compounds such as flavonoids, polyphenols, spices and others. These plant compounds are also known for they anti-oxidative capacity; hence, they seem to have a dualistic mechanism inside the cell. Exercise is another stressor that modulates the OSR pathway. Demirovic and colleagues (2014) note:

"The contraction of muscles requires large amounts of oxygen to be consumed during the oxidative phosphorylation in the mitochondria. This results in excess production of reactive oxygen species (ROS) that will trigger the OSR in the cells." [53]

The **nutritional stress response** (NSR) is activated in response to an organism's lack of nutrients. The purpose of NSR is to mediate the survival of the organism during the period of deprivation. Stressors known to activate NSR include food limitation, hypoxia (low oxygen conditions), damaged organelles, etc. Several research studies point out that at the organismic level, NSR reduces metabolism and limits reproduction, while at cellular level it increases autophagy (programmed cell death) [53, 54, 55, 56].

In my interpretation, autophagy (often known as self-eating) is a cellular maintenance and renewal mechanism whose purpose is to remove damaged proteins and cellular debris. According to Yang and Klionsky (2010), autophagy operates at basal levels (under normal conditions), but is enhanced as mTOR (amino-acid sensing pathway involved in growth) and insulin are downregulated [53, 56]:

"However, under conditions of limitation or deprivation of amino acids, growth factors, and other nutrients, or when macromolecules become damaged, aggregated, fibrillated, or in some other way modified and not used by the cells, or the cell lacks nutrients or energy, AP is enhanced." [53, 56]

Demirovic et al. (2014) are in favor of reaping the potential health benefits of NSR through practices such as calorie restriction, intermittent fasting, and periodic fasting. They argument that:

"Induction of AP and enhanced basal levels of autophagic flux on chronic or intermittent and periodic CR and fasting is the earliest and consistent molecular mechanism for clearing up the intracellular debris." [53]

The **energy stress response** (ESR) occurs in the context of reduced energy levels. Energy depletion and low energy levels are characterized by increased ratios of AMP/ATP and NAD+/NADH. Such conditions can be the result of exercise (working out), food restriction, impairment in glucose uptake, as well as increased oxidation of fatty acids. The energy stress response is mediated primarily through AMPk and sirtuins, which have been found to act synergistically [53].

AMPk (AMP-activated protein kinase) is an energy sensing molecule. It responds to low-energy levels inside the cell and its purpose is to restore energy balance. AMPk activation occurs within minutes of an energy deficient state:

"AMPK is involved in the regulation of energy metabolism by directly affecting the transcription of several genes for key metabolic pathways, especially carbohydrate and lipid metabolism, protein biosynthesis, and mitochondrial biogenesis." [53]

Sirtuins are a family of proteins that act as metabolic sensors and have been involved in influencing processes such as: stress resistance, apoptosis, transcription, mitochondria biogenesis, and inflammation, in situations of food shortage (energy depletion) and not only. Their activity is mostly dependent on the cellular NAD+/NADH ratio [57].

Unlike AMPk, the sirtuins' response occurs after a few hours of an energy deficient state and it involves processes such as: gluconeogenesis, apoptosis, oxidation of fatty acids, uptake of glucose, inflammation, and insulin secretion. Demirovic and colleagues (2014) name a few stressors to induce the energy stress response, such as: quercetin, resveratrol, different polyphenols, spices, rolipram, as well as synthetic compounds that activate sirtuins and AMPk [53].

The **DNA damage response** (DDR) is a cellular stress response to agents such as radiation, free radicals, different oxidants, ROS, and others. DNA lesions that activate DDR include: modification of DNA bases, formation of abasic sites, single strand and double strand DNA breaks (SSB, DSB) and others [53].

The response to such lesions (DDR) is the activation of numerous repair and removal/disposal mechanisms:

"These pathways include base excision repair (BER), nucleotide excision repair, non-homologous end-joining, homologous recombination, and ataxia-telangiectasia mutated (ATM)-mediated and ataxia-telangiectasiamutated and Rad3-related (ATR)-mediated DDR signaling." [53]

Jackson and Bartek (2009) consider that an optimal DNA damage response is crucial in situations like: maintaining proper telomeres, generating immune receptor diversity, appropriate cell differentiation, as well as the prevention of different diseases and pathologic conditions [58].

Demirovic et al. (2014) describe DDR in the hormesis context:

"Although health beneficial hormetic effects of various DNA damaging agents, especially radiation exposure to UV-, X-, and γ-rays, have been reported, the details of the DDR have not been well-studied." [53]

The **unfolded protein response** (UPR) is another cellular response to stressors. It is triggered by unfolded and misfolded proteins in the endoplasmic reticulum (ER). Stressors and proteotoxic agents such as hypoxia, oxidants, virus infections, and the activity of different hormones and toxic chemicals can lead to protein unfolding or misfolding in the ER lumen. Such ER stress leads to higher levels of chaperones (to assist in protein folding), higher levels of cellular clearance of debris, as well as higher anti-oxidant capacity [53].

In a 2016 paper, Zhang and colleagues showed how activating UPR in the mitochondria by administering a compound to raise NAD+ levels leads to rejuvenation of stem cells and extends lifespan in animal models [59].

It would be interesting to see the applicability or the effect of using such compounds in humans. Even though such products exist on the market, there is little human research to support their use; plus, they are still quite expensive. However, cheaper interventions such as fasting or caloric restriction may elicit similar NAD+ boosting effects.

The **inflammatory response** (ISR), the last one to be mentioned in this section, is a cellular stress response triggered by allergens, ROS, pathogens, different damaged macromolecules, and others.

Low levels of inflammation support health within organisms; on the other hand, chronic inflammation is detrimental. Many cell types are involved in the inflammation process (such as, neutrophils, monocytes, macrophages, etc) and one of their most important molecular products is the nuclear factor kappa-B (NFKB). Upon activation, NFKB controls processes such as DNA transcription, production of cytokines, as well as cell survival - and their numerous associated sub-processes. I will provide a more detailed description of this (for the geeks) later in the book.

Adaptation and Cross Resistance

Stress response is most often adaptive, that is: the organism becomes tolerant to increasing levels of perturbing agents. This can promote better survival unless the damage from the stressor is too high and leads to a pathologic condition.

Perturbing agents to induce adaptive responses in different organisms include: heat stress, oxidative stress, alkalizing agents, heavy metals, and radiation, to name a few.

As mentioned by Crawford and Davies (1994), when human lymphocytes are exposed to low level radiation from tritiated thymidine (used for labeling DNA in cell studies), they become more resistant to chromosomal damage by high doses of X-rays [60].

In the context of oxidative stress, cells use two main methods of defense:

1. By increasing the activity of anti-oxidant enzymes and molecules, such as [60]:

- superoxide dismutases (SODs)
- glutathione peroxidases
- catalase
- glutathione
- ascorbate (vitamin C)

2. By increasing the activity of repair enzymes:

"These repair systems remove and/or repair oxidatively damaged macromolecules. DNA repair often involves DNA nucleases and glycosylases." [60]

Milisav (2011) extend this bimodal view of cell stress response to a process characterized by 4 main events [61]:

1. Induction of cell repair mechanisms
2. Temporary adaptation to stressor
3. Induction of autophagy
4. Cell death

These are not necessarily interdependent. The level to which one or more of these mechanisms is activated depends on the level of stress the cell is being exposed to, as well as the frequency and the duration of exposure. When the stressor is too perturbing, the cell may not be able to induce efficient repair and/or adaptation, thus leading to cell death.

Besides the previously discussed chaperones (proteins assisting folding/unfolding of other proteins), NFKB, and other stressor molecules, a factor worth mentioning in this context of cellular response is p53. According to Milisav (2011):

"Transformation-related protein 53 (p53) is a transcription factor, which responds to many types of cellular stress, such as DNA damage, hypoxia and oncogene activation. It regulates target genes that induce cell cycle arrest, apoptosis, senescence, DNA repair or changes in metabolism." [61]

p53 is kept inactive in unstressed cells. When the cell undergoes stress, p53 levels increase leading to the transcription of numerous genes that control cell cycle and apoptosis. Often, cell cycle stops and given the levels of stress and the capacity of the cell to respond and appropriately adapt to it, the cell may lose its ability to divide, hence becoming senescent.

While p53 responds to intrinsic stress, NFKB responds to extrinsic stress (from the outside of the cells). These mechanisms cannot run simultaneously within a cell. When one is activated, the other is inactivated.

Acclimation, or physiologic adjustment, that leads to increased tolerance of stress is a conserved mechanism that has been observed across all specters of life: from bacteria to multicellular organisms and to humans. Acclimation is the result of the adaptive response to stress.

When a normal cell is subjected to a stressor that it cannot handle, it dies. If the stressor is provided at sub lethal doses, the normal cell becomes a stressed cell that undergoes an adaptive response:

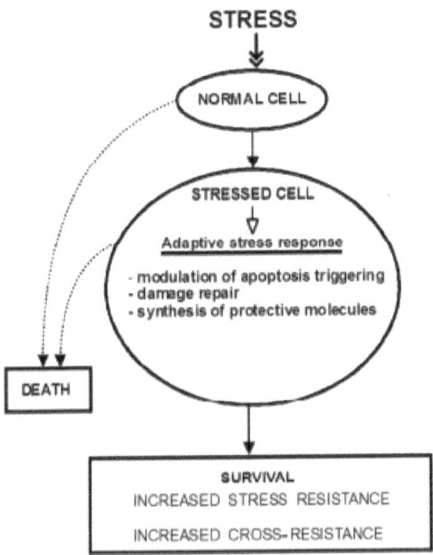

Adaptive Stress Response. Adapted from Milisav and colleagues (2012) [62]

The three main mechanisms of adaptive response, according to Milisav et al. (2012), are: modulation of apoptosis, damage repair, and induction of cytoprotective molecules [62].

Another important factor in adaptive stress is mTORC1 (mammalian target of rapamycin complex I); it is a cellular energy/nutrient sensor that controls protein synthesis. Activated by amino acids, it leads to higher protein and lipid synthesis and increased energy metabolism. Inhibited by hypoxia, genotoxic stress (genome damage), and energy deficits, it leads to increased autophagy and lysosome biogenesis.

Adaptive response is, in my opinion, desirable. For it to occur, the levels at which the stressors are being delivered is of importance. Previously mentioned stressors including radiation, oxidants, phytochemicals, heat shock, dietary restriction, ischemia, hypergravity, exercise and others have been shown to induce cross resistance, aside of stress resistance.

In my own definition, cross resistance is the ability of a cell or organisms to withstand perturbation from a second stressor upon the exposure to an initial different stressor. For example, cells exposed to heat stress develop tolerance (cross-resistance) to cyanide exposure. Here are a few more examples of cross resistance [62]:

Cells **exposed to hydrogen peroxide** (H_2O_2) develop cross resistance to heat shock, gamma and X-ray radiation.

Cells **exposed to heat shock** develop resistance to H_2O_2 and cyanide (as seen above) and they also show a delay in aging. Heat shock responses include the overexpression of heat shock proteins (HSP) which can lead to increased levels of glutathione, thus conferring protection against subsequent oxidative stress.

Fruit flies **exposed to cold** develop resistance to heat shock and they also show an increase in lifespan.

When cells are **exposed to toxic chemicals** and agents such as DNP (2,4 dinitrophenol) they become more tolerant to ischemia [62]. As per Milisav and colleagues (2012):

"Recent findings imply that health benefits of many phytochemicals may be the consequence of cross-resistance in which a phytochemical activates one or more adaptive stress response pathways. Beneficial effects for health have been demonstrated for many chemicals isolated from plants." [62]

When rat cells are **stressed by exercise** they become more tolerant to heat stress and ischemia.

When humans are **stressed by exercise** they develop tolerance to ischemia and they show a delay in aging.

Caloric restriction increases tolerance, across all walks of life - from simple cells to humans, - go lower temperature, heat stress, H2O2 and they show a delay in the aging process:

"Globally, the effects of CR are achieved through modulating the IGF1/insulin and mTOR signaling pathways, gene expression regulation, including through DNA methylation and histone acetylation/deacetylation." [62]

Hypergravity occurs when the force of gravity is higher than the gravity levels on the ground. Subjects exposed to higher G loads may have to adapt to bearing higher weights (think of weight lifting). Higher loads may increase the metabolic demand on the subject, which may increase oxidative stress and ROS production, thus inducing a more active anti-oxidant system. Milisav and colleagues (2012) report that these hypergravity induced cross tolerance effects have been observed mostly in animal models; I would suspect the situation is not much different in humans. We can see the effects of weigh bearing exercise on muscle strength and growth in people who lift weights frequently.

Adaptive response to stress is beneficial and desirable. However, very high levels of stressors delivered in a short period of time, as well as chronic exposure to stress (without allowing the organism to respond adaptively) can be harmful and disease promoting.

To complicate things a bit further, not all low-dose exposures to stressors are beneficial; a reason to be skeptic about the widely applicable (generalized) mechanisms of hormesis that are proposed by Calabrese and others.

As Hadley (2003) points out, *"low doses of a tumour suppressor can actually promote tumour growth, and small amounts of various bactericides can promote bacterial colony growth."* [63]. I think it is safe to say that low dose exposure to stressors can be beneficial, but not all low dose exposure to stressors are actually beneficial; which is why every strategy must be carefully contextualized and individually built. Let us now briefly turn to mechanisms of disease resistance triggered by exposure to stressors via adaptive cell stress response pathways.

Disease Resistance through ACSRP

To be able to cope with the hostile conditions of primitive Earth, cells had to adopt mechanisms of protection against ROS, large temperature fluctuations, UV light, and unfavorable pH, to name a few. As per Mattson (2008), evolution is in favor of organisms that can use environmental toxic agents in their favor. Such toxic factors often serve as signaling molecules that induce adaptive stress responses. Carbon monoxide, nitric oxide, glutamate, TNF-alpha, calcium and potassium ions are some examples [64].

In higher organisms, similar factors can come in the form of caloric restriction, vigorous exercise, intake of plant phytochemicals, intermittent and prolonged fasting. If such stressors elicit appropriate adaptive responses, this can lead to protection against cardiovascular disease, diabetes, some types of cancers, and can extend healthy lifespan.

If the dose of the stressor is modulated appropriately, it can also elicit positive cognitive adaptations. Mattson (2008) likes to call this as 'neurohormesis'. I have trouble with the pronunciation of that word. Why not use more simple words like 'cognitive stress tolerance' which can be understood word-by-word by the lay public? Here's how he thinks it works [64]:

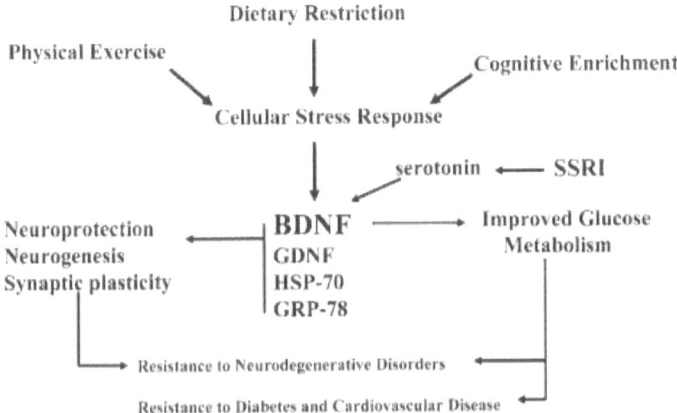

Cognitive benefits from certain stressors. Adapted from Mattson (2008) [64]

Following the logic, such a mechanism can prevent neuron degeneration that occurs in the normal aging process, thus promoting long-term cognitive health. An increase in BDNF (brain derived neurotrophic factor) may lead to enhanced learning and memory via the production of new neural cells.

Similarly, when the brain is exposed to low oxygen conditions (a stressor), the adaptive response can induce tolerance to more severe hypoxia (such as in myocardial infarction or stroke) [64].

Glutamate is another factor to elicit different responses, dependent of the concentration (dose). Glutamate is the major excitatory neurotransmitter.

At low concentration, it promotes normal synaptic activity: transient calcium influx => maintenance of function. [64]

At medium concentration, it elicits a cognitive stimulatory effect (often characterized by mild ischemia): moderately transient calcium influx => stress response => enhanced function. [64]

High levels of glutamate can induce seizures and severe ischemia: sustained calcium influx (toxicity) => cell dysfunction and death. [64]

Once again, I have to mention the importance of appropriately modulating the dose of the stressor. And as pointed by Mattson (2008), inducing stress resistance mechanisms via dietary, behavioral and toxin-based strategies can hold promise for preventing and treating a wide spectrum of diseases, including diabetes, cardiovascular diseases, cancer, and neurodegeneration.

At this point, you have reached a good level of familiarity with the mechanisms of stressors and physiologic stress. In the next part of the book, I will focus on specific situations where stress and stressors can benefit human health. Some of the topics include: exercise, diet, fasting, temperature stress, cognitive stress, and radiation. I will often provide anecdotal examples from my personal experiences.

Chapter 3:
Exercise Physiology - Stress and Adaptation

In this chapter I aim to explore how positive stress (eustress) can be integrated into exercise physiology to build strength and muscle mass and, more indirectly, for weight loss. In my current view, I do not think that exercise alone is a powerful weight loss tool, in light of what I've seen from research and from the personal reports of other people. Simply put, exercise as a primary strategy for weight loss seems to fail when other lifestyle factors - one of the most important, diet - are not attributed appropriate consideration.

I do not wish to find any rigid exercising routine (a gold standard, if I may) that would be followed indefinitely for the purposes of strength gain and weight loss. Rather, my goal is to find a combination of strategies to be used cyclically or, even better, a strategy that is adapted consistently.

I derive my inspiration from the works of numerous exercise physiologists and researchers who are in favor of periodized strategies. Personally, I began implementing periodization in my weight lifting workouts not so very long ago. Thus, I will make anecdotal reports whenever is appropriate. Before getting into the 'meat' of this topic, let me briefly introduce an anti-thesis of a health promoting lifestyle in the context of exercise.

The Couch Potato

According Mattson and Calabrese (2009), when the cells of the body are unchallenged, they become more vulnerable to injury and disease. Too much food intake and too little physical exercise can result in insulin resistance, which in time can promote the development of diabetes and other conditions of the metabolic syndrome. A couch potato is then exemplified as follows [2]:

"The extreme example of an unhealthy lifestyle is the person who gets no exercise, eats excessive amounts of high-calorie foods, and avoids intellectually challenging tasks." [2]

A while ago I used to believe that a healthy life depends on many more factors additional to diet and exercise; factors related to electromagnetic field radiation and its effects on the human body, factors related to supplementation, and other factors lacking strong and rigorous support from the scientific community. I used to believe in a flawed theory that does not promote the fact that weight loss is mostly dependent on how much you eat and how much energy you spend. I used to believe in fantastic theories - that caloric intake does not matter when following nutrition protocols like the ketogenic diet.

But as I read more scientific studies and as I continued altering many different variables in my lifestyle, I learned that diet and exercise are probably the biggest and most important factors to a healthy life; sleep is as important; I know that sounds boring...

To lose weight, you'd have to restrict calories to allow your body to match its energy needs from endogenous sources (from within the body; think of the adipose tissue). Your resting metabolic rate (RMR) and your daily energy requirements (TEE - total energy expenditure) are variables. They fluctuate consistently; thus getting a baseline value may be tricky, if that is even possible. Losing weight becomes a matter of constantly monitoring and adjusting these and other variables. If you plateau (with weight loss) when you are following a calorically restricted diet, it probably means your body's metabolic rate has adjusted and you may have to adjust your strategy accordingly.

When you are in an energy deficit from eating fewer calories and/or more exercise, cells in your body succumb to a slight metabolic stress. They respond adaptively by increasing insulin sensitivity (on one hand), allowing them to be more receptive to glucose, by increasing their energy reliance on fat, and by upregulating the production of other hormones and cytokines responsible for adaptive stress response.

Similar to physiologic challenges through diet and exercise, cognitive challenges provoke mild neuronal stress. Such stress can influence neuronal Na+ and Ca2+ influx, leading to higher energy production (more ATP and more NAD+) and increased free radical production [2]. Increased oxidative stress may activate the Nrf2-ARE pathway, resulting in the production of proteins that confer protection against oxidative stress, such as: heme oxygenase-1 and NQO1 (an oxidoreductase). In this way, cognitive challenges may increase the ability of neurons to deal with Ca2+ influx and with higher oxidative and metabolic stress.

These neuronal and peripheral (in other parts of the body, outside the brain) adaptations may be induced through frequent exercise. Caloric restriction and cognitive challenges may allow for additive effects, if they are implemented together. Exercise can be of many types, depending on the energy system it relies on.

Endurance exercise may increase oxidative metabolism by relying on the TCA cycle for energy production, while intense resistance exercise may rely more on the ATP-CP pathway and on glycolysis. These are two extremes of the exercise spectrum. Variations between and beyond these two are numerous. The one that I'm going to focus on in this chapter is resistance training. I want to sketch ways for how it can be implemented strategically to provide as many health benefits as possible, mostly in terms of strength and muscle gains, but also for its cognitive benefits.

Resistance Training - Important Variables

Think of resistance training as being a type of physical activity in which muscle or a muscle group is exercised against external resistance. The classical example is weight lifting, in which the trainee works with free weights (barbells, dumbells, kettlebells, other weights) or machines (leg press machine, chest press machine, curl machines, etc). Lighter loads, medium loads, and heavy loads are all included in resistance training through weight lifting, which is why there are numerous protocols that you can create and follow. For example, body builders may work with moderate loads, while those who train for strongmen competitions may work with heavier loads (very roughly speaking).

When weight lifting for resistance training (and depending on your goals), there are several variables that should be considered, including, but not limited to: frequency of training, volume, type of exercise, loading, resting intervals, and intensity. I'm going to discuss the ones I consider the most important.

According to Schoenfeld (2016), **frequency of training** refers to the number of training sessions in a given period of time, most often a week. Resistance training done three times a week may lead to better body composition. However, frequency of training should not be assessed independent of other variables like intensity, volume, and loading. Sessions of higher intensity, larger volume and increased loads may require longer resting periods (days until the next session); this allows muscle damage to be repaired efficiently, thus adapting it to higher subsequent stress or perturbation [65]. Schoenfeld (2016) explains this better:

"Intense lifting results in structural damage to the muscle fibers. During recovery, the body repairs this damage so that the muscle comes back bigger and stronger for the next bout. But if you hit the same

muscle hard before the process has fully run its course, you deprive it of the opportunity to repair." [65]

Schoenfeld proposes **resting** for at least 48 hours between exercises that target the same muscle group, arguing that this is the approximate amount of time for higher protein synthesis to occur following a resistance training session [65]. Training with lighter loads and lower volume may allow for more frequent (more than 3 times per week) sessions. Heavier loads, higher intensity and a larger volume per session may require lowering the frequency of training.

Whatever frequency is selected, I propose not to follow it indefinitely. Frequency of training should be periodized for continuous strength and muscle gains. Let me exemplify this with my current personal experience.

I break down my weight training in periods of 1 week. There are weeks when I train with heavier loads (weights), fewer sets and fewer repetitions per set. During such weeks, my frequency of training is 3 times per week. There are weeks when I train with moderate loads (weights), more sets and more repetitions per sets. During such weeks, my frequency of training is 4-5 times per week. Quite often, I train with heavier and moderate loads in the same session, alternating between sets with more repetitions and moderate loads and sets with fewer repetitions and heavier loads. This is a simplistic example of periodization for the sake of your immediate understanding of the concept. My training strategy is more dynamic and ever changing. However, one of the few constants in my strategy involves the **intensity of effort**, which I purpose to maintain high, except for deloading sessions.

Schoenfeld (2016) talks about increasing frequency as the trainee gains training experience:

"This allows your body to acclimate to the heightened stress from more frequent training sessions. In the early phases, you'll use a total-body routine so that each muscle is trained multiple times per week. This enhances the neural response, facilitating your ability to hone your exercise technique. In the advanced phases, a split routine allows you to perform a greater volume while providing proper recovery between sessions." [65]

Volume is another very important variable for resistance training. There is no single prescription for manipulating volume for strength and muscle gains. As a positive stress to the body, volume has to be assessed contextually. While single set routines may promote hypertrophy, overtraining may be detrimental to hypertrophy. In-between you will find a plethora of sweet spots for optimal volume and optimal hypertrophy.

According to Schoenfeld (2016), recognized by many as a leading figure in exercise physiology, volume should be manipulated over time:

"Ideally, this is accomplished by instituting periodic high-volume training phases to promote functional overreaching. These overreaching phases should be relatively brief and involve pushing your body to its limits and then pulling back in volume and intensity so that you don't become overtrained." [65]

Do you remember the concept of adaptive homeostasis that I discussed previously? That of pushing the functional range of an organism...

In adaptive homeostasis, appropriate exposure to a stressor may expand the range within which an organism can function properly, allowing for a more flexible survival. Similarly, bouts of increasing volume and intensity over the course of a few subsequent training sessions would promote a super-compensatory response, leading to efficient muscle development.

Some might call it over-reaching; others might call it progressive overload.

Good muscle development can then be achieved, provided that enough recuperation is allowed between these bouts of high volume and high intensity training. In this case, alternating high-volume training with deloading (lower volume, lower intensity, and lighter weights) may help avoid overtraining. Thus, deloading periods are favorable for appropriate muscle repair and growth. Deloading may also resensitize the muscle, enabling it to respond adaptively to subsequent lower doses of perturbation.

Even though overtraining is a bit exaggerated, I think it exists, but it is not as prevalent as some consider. People think they are exhausted because they spend too much time in the gym working out, when the reality is that they pay much less attention to variables like nutrition and sleep, which contribute to their incapacity to handle exercise stress.

Higher cortisol secretion and lower testosterone levels are characteristic of 'real' overtraining. More importantly, overtraining may lead to muscle catabolism. Signs and symptoms of overtraining include, but are not limited to: elevated resting blood pressure and heart rate, lower appetite, lower desire to exercise and lower exercise performance.

I have experienced such symptoms. I can recall a time when I went to the gym 5 days in a row and I tried working out with the same levels of high intensity, high volume, and heavier weights. The fourth and the fifth days were forceful and very challenging mentally, not only physically. I had no desire to go to the gym and I felt like being at the limits of exertion. My biggest craving was to stay in bed and sleep.

Luckily, I did not injure myself. It took a couple of days of avoiding the gym perimeter to return my desire to workout.

When I got back, I was able to progress to heavier weights and higher volume training.

Another important factor of resistance training is **loading,** or the resistance that goes against the muscle. In weight lifting, one can train with different loads: light, moderate, heavy, and anything in between.

Lighter loads are often used by trainees who want to maintain muscular tone. I personally view it as a sort of aerobic exercise with weights. It doesn't promote adaptive responses in the muscle and it's least likely to lead to muscle and strength gains.

Moderate loads are a favorite of bodybuilders. Higher intensity and higher volume generically come within the same package. Using moderate loads may make the trainee less susceptible to injury. This type of strategy can induce muscular adaptive stress responses that promote strength and muscle gains.

Heavier loads are often used by trainees engaged in power-lifting and strongmen competitions. Fewer sets, fewer repetitions (lower volume), and lower frequency characterize this regimen of training. Working with heavier weights may increase the risk of injury compared to a bodybuilder-type routine.

When I began lifting weights, I used heavy loads and compound movements (exercises that engage multiple muscle groups). I would go to the gym 1-3 times per week, doing routines that included: squats, barbell curls, chest presses, and leg presses. I would do 1-3 sets of 5-8 repetitions per set. The entire workout would last 20-30 minutes at maximum, but it would be very intense and very taxing on the body, requiring me to allow a couple of days of rest between sessions.

Besides categorizing training load as being light, moderate, or heavy, there is a categorization based on the concept of 1 Rep-Max.

1RM is the maximum load with which a trainee can perform 1 repetition of an exercise. It is often used as a baseline for other types of training. For example, some advocates of high-intensity training promote working with 85% of 1RM - a load (weight) that is 85% of the maximum load with which one can do 1 repetition. To be more specific and to correlate lighter, moderate, and heavier loads with the concept of 1RM, let me exemplify:

- light routines - 12+ sets with 30-50% of 1RM
- moderate routines - 8-12 sets with 70-80% of 1RM
- heavy routines - 3-5 set with 85%+ of 1RM

This degree of variability allows for multiple types of training protocols that can be designed for good muscle development. The one that I currently rely most on is a bodybuilding-type routine with moderate weights, higher-volume, higher-intensity and increased frequency of training. To make it more efficient, I alternate (periodize) this routine with other protocols. Schoenfeld (2016) also discusses this type of protocol:

"The use of medium loads generates considerable metabolic stress. The associated buildup of metabolites influences growth in multiple ways, including the production of growth factors, increased cell swelling, and greater muscle fiber activation." [65]

Intensity of effort is one of the most important factors of training that I aim to keep constant. The exception is when I use deloading workouts: I train with lower weights and lower volume. In such circumstances, intensity is moderate to low.

For muscle to develop, it must be challenged beyond its capacity. According to Schoenfeld (2016):

"By nature, the human body doesn't like change. It strives to maintain stability - a phenomenon called homeostasis. Nudging your body from its homeostatic state requires progressively higher levels of effort; otherwise, it is not sufficiently challenged and thus has not impetus to adapt." [65]

The challenge, then, becomes finding the right dose of the stressor (resistance, in this case), the frequency, and the duration of exposure. Not 'nudging' your muscle beyond its limits (over-reaching), and you may fall short on achieving good muscle development. Pushing yourself too hard and too frequently, and you may end up overtraining and catabolizing your muscle. In my view, this is a never ending game of testing, observing, (failing), and optimizing.

So far, I've used weight lifting to make a case for muscle and strength development. But there are numerous other ways that work for the same purpose, examples including: bodyweight training, calisthenics, crossfit, sprinting, swimming, boxing, cycling and other types of protocols that engage type II muscle fibers, which are responsible for bulk muscle development (strength and mass).

I specifically did not mention endurance training because it does not promote higher strength and mass. Endurance training taxes type I muscle fibers, which do not lead to muscle gains but promote muscle endurance.

Endurance training can provide health benefits, as long as it is not done chronically, which can lead to the development of pathologic states. I have experienced with chronic (every-day) endurance training (jogging) in the past. But I do not have enough experience or knowledge to discuss it extensively here. That is why, for the remaining of the chapter, I will discuss muscle development mostly from a resistance training perspective.

Let us now turn to exploring strength development from a research perspective.

Strength Development in Athletes

This meta-analysis from 2004 wanted to determine optimal doses of training for maximal strength gains in athletes. Peterson and colleagues analyzed 37 studies and included the following variables in their study [66]:

- age and gender of participants,
- training frequency (days/week of training a certain muscle group),
- training intensity (% of 1RM used),
- training volume (in terms of sets completed per muscle group per workout),
- use of creatine,
- periodization of the training protocol [66].

In short, they found that maximal strength gains are obtained in athletes who train at ~85% of 1RM (intensity), twice a week (frequency), and with an average of 8 sets per muscle group (volume). They accounted for ~370 effect sizes [66].

Analyzing the dose-response curves that came out of the data, they also found that training at lower intensity (50-70% of 1RM) and lower volume (1-3 sets) leads to minimal strength gains [66]. I'd suspect that untrained athletes would still benefit from this type of protocol. More advanced athletes could gain from a protocol of lower intensity training by increasing the volume of training per workout. As per Peterson and colleagues (2004):

"Faster rates of muscular strength improvement at smaller doses of resistance training are typical during earlier periods of training or for previously untrained individuals and are likely attributed to neural adaptations resulting in enhanced motor unit activation." [66]

Athletes usually start with low-volume training. As they adapt, they may need to gradually increase the volume to continuously overload the muscular and neuromuscular systems (over-reaching) and to continuously stimulate hormonal systems to promote ongoing strength development [66].

Similar to Schoenfeld (2016) [65], these researchers point out that dosing of intensity, frequency, and volume can be considered some of the foremost disputed variables in training. In my view, modulating these variables is crucial for continuous adaptive muscular response.

While they found greater strength gains in participants who used creatine, training to failure, and periodized training protocols, they note that such variables did not significantly alter the overall dose-response trends in their data [66]. I would suspect that such variables can make a great difference in muscle development in more advanced athletes.

In conclusion, Peterson and colleagues report that their study confirms the existence of different dose-response relationships for strength gains in competitive athletes [66]. They are in favor of using the principle of progressive overload when designing optimal exercising strategies.

Before moving on to exploring the molecular mechanisms of muscle development, let us review the findings of two additional meta-analyses. I selected these papers out of a dozen initial, because I consider them examples of good research practices. I am confident that there are countless of other good or better studies in the literature. Searching for and interpreting them would limit/narrow the purpose of this book.

I'd welcome you to exercise good critical thinking skills, do not take my interpretations of these studies for granted, do not take these studies for granted, ask yourself why they may not be good studies, and conduct your personal search on the topic, should it be of your interest. I will keep making this suggestion throughout the book. Now, let us delve into these meta-analyses.

In a 2016 meta-analysis, Lesinski, Prieske and Granacher examined dose-response relationships of resistance training on physical performance in young athletes. This study was published in the *British Journal of Sports Medicine* [67].

They initially identified 576 potential studies for their analysis, out of which only 43 made it into the quantitative analysis. 1558 athletes were included in the analysis: 891 of them doing resistance training (RT) in 62 intervention groups:

RT interventions: between 4 and 80 weeks
Frequency of training: between 1 and 3 sessions per week
Volume: 1-8 sets/exercise, 4-15 reps/set
Rest intervals: 20-220 seconds between sets
Intensity: between 35% and 88% of 1RM

According to Lesinski et al. (2016):

"Subgroup analyses demonstrated that different training types of RT produced significantly different gains in muscle strength ($p<0.001$), agility ($p<0.05$) and sport-specific performance ($p<0.05$)." [67]

Training with free weights lead to larger effects on agility and muscle strength. Sport-specific performance (these were athletes engaged in different sports) was achieved with more complex training - combination of training protocols.

Dose response relationships for RT parameters suggest the most effective interventions to improve strength are [67]:

RT intervention: > 23 weeks
Volume: 5 sets/exercise, 6-8 reps/set
Intensity: 80-89% of 1RM
Rest interval: 3-4 min between sets.

Reading the entire study will allow you to see the effects that each different dose of training variable elicited on muscle strength development.

Researchers pointed out that both volume and intensity have to be carefully considered when prescribing resistance training for maximal physiologic adaptations and minimal risk of injury. They are in favor of fewer repetitions and higher intensity. I'd add that fewer repetitions per set do not necessarily translate into fewer sets of an exercise per session of training. Thus, this could also turn into a protocol of moderate-to-high volume and higher intensity of training. No matter the protocol used, it should not be followed indefinitely and in a fixated manner (rigidly). According to Lesinski and colleagues (2016):

"Different configurations of training volume and intensity result in different forms of physiological stress, which in turn induce different neural and muscular adaptations." [67]

They are also careful to point out some of the limitations in their analysis:

"Further limitations of this systematic review and meta-analysis are the high risk of bias of the included studies (only 4 out of 43 studies reached a PEDro score of≥6), the considerable heterogeneity between studies (ie, I^2=41–81%), and the uneven distribution of SMDs calculated for the respective training parameters." [67]

The PEDro scale represents a measure of methodological quality in clinical trials. To learn more about it, see these references [69, 70]. I would also add that to define good exercise protocols, one must analyze or conduct studies in non-homogenous cohorts (healthy - athletes, lifters, sedentary, etc - and non-healthy) with different interventions including not only resistance training, but a whole host of other training protocols. With these in mind, I consider this meta-analysis itself as a reflection of good methodology. Let us now look into the findings of another meta-analysis.

Published in 2003, this meta-analysis purposed to determine the dose-response relationship for strength development so that proper training protocols can be prescribed for strength gains [68]. Rhea and colleagues included 140 studies with a total of 1433 effect sizes in their analysis.

Even though they had many studies in the analysis, the sample size per intervention was small, which is why researchers acknowledged that their findings may have low statistical power. Additionally, they had 21 studies with subjects of 55 years or older, 13 studies with competitive athletes, and 6 studies with subjects younger than 18 years [68]. Hence, we can derive important insights from this analysis given its magnitude, but we should examine additional evidence to make sure that whatever strategy we choose, we have solid evidence to support it. What they found [68]:

Intensity

- untrained subjects (<1 year of training) - maximal strength gains at 60% 1RM (or ~12 reps with 60% of 1RM)
- trained subjects - maximal strength gains at 80% 1RM (or ~8 reps with 80% of 1RM)

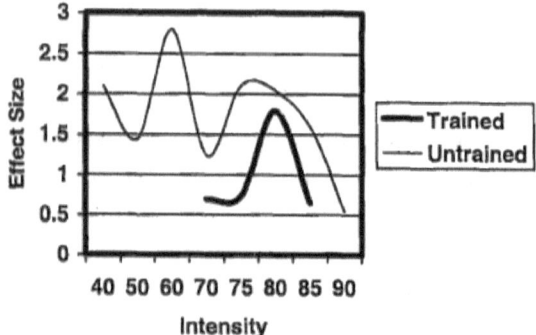

FIGURE 1—Dose-response curves for intensity.

Adapted from Rhea et al. (2003) [68]

Frequency

- untrained subjects - maximal gains when training for 3 days/week/muscle group
- trained subjects - maximal gains when training for 2 days/week/muscle group

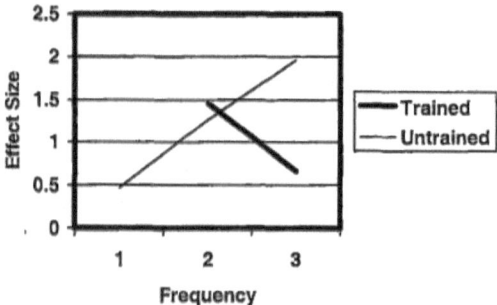

FIGURE 2—Dose-response curves for frequency.

Adapted from Rhea et al. (2003) [68]

Volume

- trained and untrained subjects - max. gains at ~4 sets/muscle group

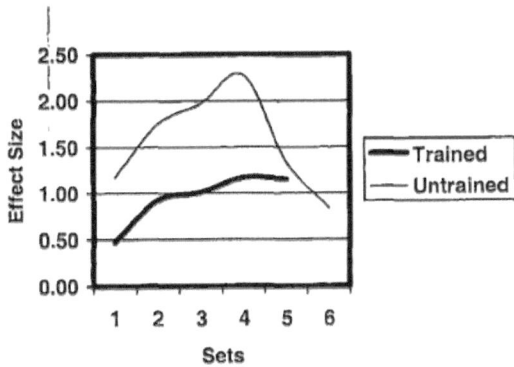

FIGURE 3—Dose-response curves for volume.

Adapted from Rhea et al. (2003) [68]

With the findings from their analysis, Rhea and colleagues (2003) were not able to support findings from previous research studies, such as that [68]:

- healthy, untrained adults - no significant benefits from multiple set protocols in their initial training period compared to single-set protocols
- single-set protocols in recreationally trained individuals will continue to elicit similar strength benefits like in multiple-set protocols

As they point out [68]:

"The magnitude of treatment effects from the 140 studies reviewed in this analysis fails to support either of these conclusions." [68]

On another note, they are in favor of the progressive overload principle by saying that:

"...such a principle is a vital characteristic in training programs of extended periods as the adaptive processes will only respond when faced with a stress to which they are not accustomed." [68]

While untrained individuals may benefit from strength gains at multiple intensities and different frequencies, as one becomes adapted to strength training, they may have to modify their protocols in such a way that they continuously exert stress on the muscle. Periodized training, variation and progressive overload are in support of such goals:

"The ACSM position statement on progression models addressed this confusion, suggesting the necessity of progressive increases in volume, intensity, and frequency of training to facilitate the adaptive processes." [68]

Rhea et al. (2003) highlight that their analysis included periodized training protocols and that even though maximal gains were observed at an average of 4 sets at 80% 1RM, subjects were training at a variety of intensities and training volumes.

"Therefore, the dose response curves presented here represent mean training levels and should not be construed as supporting training at a particular volume or intensity on a constant basis." [68]

They are in favor of effective training programs which incorporate variations in frequency, volume, and intensity - in accordance to the degree of desired strength gains.

From what I see in these meta-analysis and in other research studies in exercise physiology and from what I've experienced myself, I am in line with the fact that continuous muscle development is achieved with periodization, variation in important variables (volume, intensity, frequency, rest intervals, etc), and with applying the principle of progressive overload. Such protocols elicit continuous stress on the muscle, which is very important for adaptive responses to occur. Rigid protocols are not in support of such adaptive responses and may not favor continuous muscle development.

What we have analyzed here is just a very small and inconclusive part of the literature on exercise physiology. There are many areas requiring further exploration, such as:

- other types of exercise protocols - different from strength training,
- exercise in healthy vs. unhealthy subjects,
- exercise in lean vs. overweight and obese subjects,
- the impact of exercise in disease treatment,
- exercise in young vs. elder subjects,
- and many other similar topics.

The purpose of this book is not to discuss all of these types of exercises and their effects at length, but I suspect that the mechanisms of stress and adaptive responses play an important role in them as well. I used strength training because this is what I'm most familiar with, both from an experiential and from a research perspective. Next, I am going to succinctly go into the molecular mechanisms of muscle development.

Mechanisms of Muscle Development

Brad Schoenfeld (2010) presents a comprehensible description of how muscle develops [71]:

1. When skeletal muscle is acted upon with an overload stimulus => perturbations in myofibers and ECM (extra-cellular matrix) =>
2. This causes myogenic events => growth in the size and number of actin and myosin fibers, and increase in the number of sarcomeres =>
3. Increased diameter of individual fibers => increased muscle cross-sectional area.

Muscle, as a tissue, is not subject to significant cell replacement throughout life (compared to other tissues like skin or the lining of the gut, which are replaced often). It is a post-mitotic tissue and it is more subjected to repair than replacement.

When mechanical stimulus acts on the muscle, myogenic stem cells are activated. Most myogenic stem cells are of the type of satellite cells. When they are stimulated, these satellite cells proliferate and migrate to existing cells. Their purpose is to create new muscle fibers. They serve as the precursors needed for repairing the damaged muscle and for the subsequent growth of new muscle tissue [71].

According to Toigo and Boutellier (2006), muscle fibers can adapt to conditions of altered demand by growing longitudinally and radially, and by the regulation of fiber-type gene expression [72]. An example of a condition of altered demand is resistance training, which perturbs the tensional integrity of the muscle. Thus, resistance training can be seen as a stimulus for muscle adaptation. Such an adaptive response can be graphically depicted in the following way:

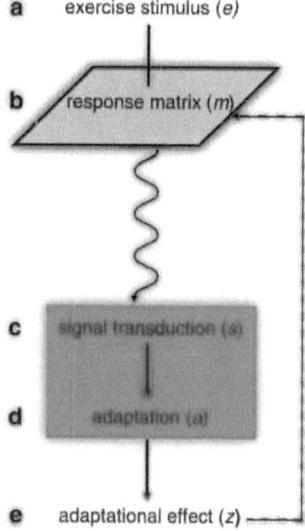

Adapted from Toigo and Boutellier (2006) [72]

This is in Toigo and Boutellier's (2006) view a simplified version of muscle perturbations being transduced into associated adaptive effects. These authors extend the category of variables that have an impact on muscle growth. They think these variables should be clearly defined when designing resistance training strategies. Additionally to volume, intensity, rest intervals, and frequency, which they categorize as classical descriptors, they add a new set of descriptors, such as:

- fractional and temporal distribution of the contraction
- modes per repetition and duration [sec] of one repetition
- rest in-between reps
- time under tension (TUT)
- volitional muscular failure
- range of motion
- recovery time in-between exercise sessions
- anatomical definition of the exercise (exercise form) [72].

While such variables may be of minor advantage for inexperienced individuals, these new descriptors can make a real difference (I suspect) when designing advanced training protocols for experienced trainees. Here's how they describe a positive adaptive case of resistance training:

"The high-intensity-short-duration workloads placed on skeletal muscle during resistance exercise are at or near maximal capacity, and as such produce significant perturbations to the skeletal muscle fibres and the associated extracellular matrix." [72]

Such perturbations can result in extensive muscle damage, especially if the trainee uses eccentric exercise (lengthening contractions) with higher loads [72]. In my opinion, this would be a good variation of a resistance training session in the repertoire of an advanced trainee. Important to keep in mind though is that muscle hypertrophy induced by resistance training occurs when muscle protein synthesis (MPS) is greater than muscle protein degradation. Toigo and Boutellier (2006) go into extensive detail describing and graphically showing how this occurs [72].

Moving from a mechanical perspective toward a molecular perspective of muscle development, numerous pathways, cellular factors and hormones are worthy to be discussed. These include: Akt/mTOR, IIS, MAPk, IGF-1, insulin, testosterone, growth hormone, and cortisol:

Akt/mTOR - master skeletal muscle growth regulator

- upon activation (phosphorylation), Akt signals mTOR => downstream effects => muscle hypertrophy
- activated Akt inhibits catabolism
- activation of Akt is mediated by IGF-1/PI3K pathway, which is triggered by increased muscle loading [72].

MAPk - Mitogen-activated protein kinase

- regulates redox status and gene expression
- specific to muscular hypertrophy - it links cellular stress with myocyte adaptive response [71].

IGF-1 - considered one of the most important anabolic hormones

According to Schoenfeld (2010), *"it is thought to provide the main anabolic response for the body as a whole and shows enhanced effects in response to mechanical loading."* [71]

During exercise, muscles produce more IGF-1 compared to the liver. They also use more IGF-1 from circulation. How much IGF-1 is available to muscles is controlled by binding proteins, IGFBPs. IGF-1 is a two-edged sword in my opinion: it can lead to indiscriminate growth: it is thought to play a central role not only in muscle hypertrophy, but also in the proliferation of tumors.

Testosterone - anabolic hormone

- similar to IGF-1, circulating testosterone is, in part, bind to SHBG. How much of it is bind is a matter of internal regulatory feedback mechanisms. Bound testosterone cannot exert its activity:

1. Unbound (not bound to SHBG) testosterone binds to androgen receptors in the cytoplasm of cells.
2. Conformational change => testosterone is carried inside the nucleus, where it directly interacts with DNA (mediating transcription processes).

According to Schoenfeld (2010), *"although the effects of testosterone on muscle are seen in the absence of exercise, its actions are magnified by mechanical loading, promoting anabolism both by increasing the protein synthetic rate and inhibiting protein breakdown."* [71]

Growth Hormone (GH)

- influences fat metabolism => mobilizing TAGs (triglycerides)
- influences amino-acid uptake into the muscle
- in the context of intense exercise, GH is associated with higher IGF-1 gene regulation in the muscle. The two factors act synergistically. [71]

Crewther and colleagues (2006) created a tabular view of these hormones and their effects on hypertrophy and power adaptations. Their analysis is based on data from multiple studies [74]:

Table III. Summary of research examining the acute anabolic and catabolic hormone responses to hypertrophy, neuronal and dynamic power schemes

	Hypertrophy	Neuronal	Dynamic power
Testosterone	↑↑↑↑	↑↑	↑↑↑↑
GH	↑↑↑↑↑↑↑↑	↑	↔
IGF-1	↑↑↑	↑↑↑↑	↔
Insulin	↔	↔	↔
Cortisol	↑↑↑↑↑	↔	↑↑

GH = growth hormone; **IGF-1** = insulin growth-like factor 1; ↑ indicates increase, ↔ indicates no change or equivocal results.

Adapted from Crewther, Cronin ad Keogh (2006) [74]

Another important aspect of muscle development involves **amino acid consumption**. In their study on the control of the size of human muscle mass, Rennie et al. (2004) noted:

"These and other recent data make a powerful point: The amount of amino acids necessary to stimulate MPS in the resting state and after exercise is in fact small (<10 g) compared with the accepted whole-body protein requirements (>70 g for most men)." [73]

Moreover:

"It has long been known that regularly active muscle is able to maximize its mass despite a poor dietary protein intake; for example, hypertrophy of a muscle can occur after the ablation of a synergist muscle even in an undernourished animal." [73]

In their narrative, Rennie and colleagues (2004) support the association of muscle hypertrophy with higher muscle protein synthesis (MPS) and adaptive increase in muscle protein breakdown:

"Of course, during the upward swing of muscle mass, MPS has to exceed MPB, and this usually requires amino acids, either dietary or possibly those diverted from other body tissues." [73]

Studying biochemistry may reveal mechanisms under which amino acids can be derived from endogenous resources, in the contexts of muscle hypertrophy (MPS > MPB) and dietary restriction.

Anecdotally, my best training (lifting) sessions have been done in the fasted state (>18-20 hours fasted). Often, I do not consume food for hours following a strenuous session, thus further prolonging my fasting. From what I can tell, I have not personally experienced negative effects because of this. Moreover, when I train fasted, and extend the fast for hours post-workout, my mental performance seems to be higher - judged by my ability to write and do mental work in a more focused and unperturbed way. I suspect that lactate may be partially responsible for this effect.

Before moving on, I want to reiterate on how resistance exercise leads to muscle adaptive responses [72]:

1. Exercise => myotrauma.
2. Activation of satellite cells through:
    - the release of anabolic cytokines from perturbed ECM (extracellular matrix)
    - inflammatory response
    - damaged myofibers
    - by satellite cells themselves (autocrine manner).
3. Upon activation, satellite cells proliferate, fuse (to existing muscle fibers or among themselves) and lead to muscle repair and/or regeneration.
4. Successful repair and regeneration are time-dependent processes:

    - if RT sessions are very frequent => prevail of degenerative processes and muscle loss.
    - if RT sessions are timed appropriately => prevail of regenerative processes and muscle gains.

With this relatively complex view of muscle development, you will have a better understanding of what I am going to discuss next: specialized routines and training protocols for advanced trainees. While using creatine, progressive overload, periodization and other specialized routines may not make much of a difference in untrained athletes (they experience muscle gains without using specialized training, especially when they just start out), I think they play an important role in more advanced athletes.

Specialized Training Routines

There are numerous techniques that can be included in the repertoire of special training routines, often implemented by high-level athletes and strength trainees. Their purpose is to promote continuous muscle development, which may be slowed-down or halted in trainees who reach a certain level of muscle development. According to Schoenfeld (2011), specialized training routines can include: drop sets, forced repetitions, heavy negatives, and supersets [75]. Let's briefly describe them:

Drop sets:

1. Perform a set to failure with a certain load
2. Reduce the load, perform another set to failure
3. Continue for as long as possible

Forced reps:

- when training with a fixed load (% of 1RM) and a fixed number of repetitions per set, when you reach your final repetition, force yourself to complete extra reps, even though you may not perform them correctly. When controlled for volume, forced reps can increase post-workout growth hormone levels [75].

Heavy negatives:

Broadly speaking, there are 3 major types of repetitions: eccentric, concentric, and isometric. Let's assume you perform a bicep curl repetition. An eccentric movement is the lengthening (or stretching) part of your repetition while a concentric movement is the shortening (or contracting) part of the movement. Isometric contraction implies no movement: the muscle contracts but it is not shortened. Imagine holding the load still at a certain angle. Here's a better way to understand the entire concept:

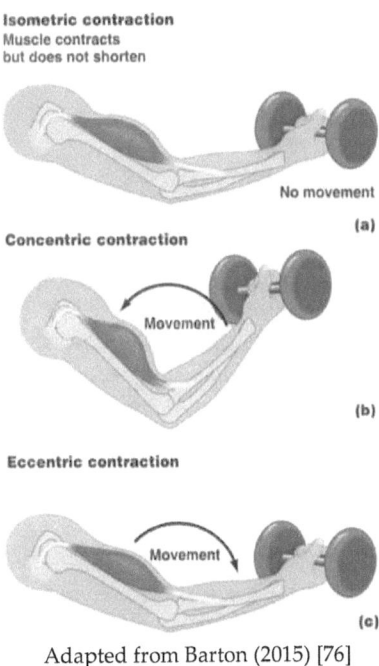

Adapted from Barton (2015) [76]

Heavy negatives, according to Schoenfeld (2011), are supramaximal loaded eccentric actions. They usually require performing eccentric contraction at loads greater than the concentric part of the repetition and they often require a spotter - person to assist. Another variation of heavy negatives is to perform the eccentric contraction slower than the concentric one - thus, focusing on the negative (eccentric is 'negative', concentric is 'positive'). Schoenfeld (2011) provides references to studies reporting how eccentric exercise can elicit greater muscle gains compared to concentric and isometric contractions [75].

Supersets:

Performing two exercises in immediate succession, thus minimizing rest intervals, is usually known as a superset. Any two exercises can be used for supersets. This type of training may make sense for further muscle development in advanced trainees because reducing rest intervals and prolonging muscle tension (by exercise) leads to higher metabolic stress and more muscular fatigue - a requirement for hypertrophy [75].

According to Schoenfeld (2011):

"These techniques should be considered advanced training strategies. Their use has a taxing effect on the neuromuscular system that is likely to exceed a beginner's capacity for adaptation. Based on the author's experience, a minimum of several months of regimented training is warranted before integrating the techniques into a routine." [75]

Periodization

Aside of the specialized techniques mentioned previously, I want to provide particular attention to periodization. I think it is beneficial in delivering efficient doses of muscle stress for continuous muscle development.

Periodization simply means a planned change in training variables, with emphasis on frequency, volume, and intensity. Periodization can be linear or non-linear, the major difference between the two being that in non-linear periodization, planned changes occur more frequently.

According to Fleck (2011), periodization in resistance training leads to higher strength gains compared to non-periodized routines [77]. Moreover:

"While both linear and nonlinear periodization plans result in significant strength and fitness gains some research indicates greater strength gains with daily nonlinear periodization." [77]

The typical planned changes involved in periodized resistance training are:

- changing the number of sets and reps (volume)
- changing the load/weight (intensity)
- changing the no. of training sessions/day or week (frequency)
- changing the resting intervals
- changing the order of exercises
- changing the type of exercise.

One may see how periodized training can easily integrate with specialized protocols, such as the ones mentioned above (forced reps, supersets, heavy negatives, etc).

In my current workout protocols I almost always combine periodized training with special routines. Basically, every RT session is different. Here are a few of the variations I use:

1. Sessions when I start with compound movements (heavy loads, fewer reps, high intensity, medium resting intervals) and I focus on eccentric contractions and finish with isolated movements (medium loads, more reps, high intensity, shorter resting

intervals); I often implement drop sets and supersets in these sessions.

2. Sessions when I only focus on compound movements and try to integrate the specialized training routines all together.

3. Sessions when I only integrate isolated movements with specialized routines.

4. Deloading sessions.

5. Sessions when I don't use specialized routines and I train like in a normal weekly split (1-3 muscle groups/session).

The main constant that I try to remain consistent with is intensity, which I aim to keep high in almost all sessions, excluding deloading sessions. In my current opinion, intensity is very important to muscle development and it can be implemented in almost all types of training regimens.

In support of periodized training, Schoenfeld and colleagues (2016) report:

"Training with a variety of repetition ranges has been theorized to provide an optimal hypertrophic stimulus to both type I and II fibers, and possibly augment the hypertrophic response as compared to training in fixed repetition ranges in isolation. The present results suggest that comparable hypertrophic, strength, and endurance adaptations occur when a varied training protocol is compared against a fixed loading program at 8–12 RM." [78]

An example of typical periodized training protocol is provided by Schoenfeld (2010) [71]:

- multiple sets with split training => higher anabolic milieu
- some sets to failure for concentric movements
- alternating training to failure with not-training to failure => avoidance of overtraining
- concentric reps carried at speeds of 1-3 seconds (fast)
- eccentric reps carried at speeds of 2-4 seconds (slower)

Moreover, Schoenfeld (2010) recommends that:

"Training should be periodized so that the hypertrophy phase culminates in a brief period of higher volume overreaching followed by a taper to allow for optimal super compensation of muscle tissue." [71]

With respect to endurance exercise, Schoenfeld et al. (2016) are careful to point out that endurance exercise may benefit from protocols with high repetitions [78]. This is one of the reasons I say that here I'm only focusing on strength and resistance training and their benefits for muscle development, while the field of exercise physiology is inclusive of many more types of exercising, in different types of subjects (healthy, sick, young, elder, etc) and for different purposes (endurance, hypertrophy, general health benefits, longevity, etc).

Side note:

Please acknowledge the narrowness of my approach and please make sure you understand that, by all means, I do not make general recommendations here. Should there be any recommendation to make to someone, I would first have to make a careful assessment of the numerous factors in that person's life; and that would turn into a very contextual and unique strategy.

In the next and last part of this chapter, I will discuss the health benefits of exercise, other than muscle development; I keep my emphasis on the mechanisms of stress and adaptation.

Health Benefits of Exercise Stressors

When we engage in physical exercise we perturb homeostasis - the inner equilibrium of the body. Such perturbations or stressors can be: mechanical, metabolic, thermal, oxidative, and hypoxic. The body responds by releasing reactive oxygen species, reactive nitrogen species, growth factors, eicosanoids and cytokines that lead to the activation of pathways involved in adaptive responses [79].

To understand how higher exercise performance and rapid recovery work, Peake and colleagues (2015) decided to analyze the scientific basis for using strategies such as antioxidant supplementation, cryotherapy, mechanical preloading, NSAIDs, heat stress, carbohydrate restriction, and blood flow restriction. They wanted to determine the involvement of such strategies in the adaptive response [79]. Here, I will discuss a few of their findings.

Carbohydrate restriction:

Modulating muscle glycogen with carbohydrate restriction can promote metabolic adaptation in the following way:

1. Strenuous exercise => higher ATP demand
2. In low glycogen conditions, this leads to higher AMPk activity
3. AMPk regulates: glucose transport, mitochondrial biogenesis and fatty acid uptake (to name a few)
4. The lower pre-exercise muscle glycogen => the higher muscle AMPk response

This can have a dual effect on protein turnover:

"In principle, higher AMPK activity (resulting from low muscle glycogen content) could attenuate muscle protein synthesis by inhibiting translation/elongation. Increased metabolic stress associated with low muscle glycogen content may also exacerbate protein degradation." [79]

Peake et al. (2015) discuss studies of different findings. One study of resistance exercise done in the context of low muscle glycogen had no effect on myofibrillar protein synthesis, while other studies have reported that exercising with low muscle glycogen leads to higher protein oxidation and degradation.

I assume that the ability to increase fatty acid oxidation during exercise can have an impact on how glycogen modulation with carbohydrate restriction affects metabolic responses. Volek and colleagues (2016) analyzed the exercise response of ultra-endurance athletes. Some of these athletes were adapted to a higher carbohydrate diet while others have been adapted to a carbohydrate restricted diet [81]. In short, the study reports that:

"Despite these marked differences in fuel use between LC and HC athletes, there were no significant differences in resting muscle glycogen and the level of depletion after 180 min of running (−64% from pre-exercise) and 120 min of recovery (−36% from pre-exercise).

Compared to highly trained ultra-endurance athletes consuming an HC diet, long-term keto-adaptation results in extraordinarily high rates of fat oxidation, whereas muscle glycogen utilization and repletion patterns during and after a 3 hour run are similar." [81]

I think it's safe to say that there is no consensus about this. Even though carbohydrate restriction and glycogen modulation can affect metabolic adaptive stress responses to exercise, the degree of impact can vary according to the characteristics of the athlete in question (age, adaptation to a certain diet, metabolic flexibility, etc). In any case, if there is a biphasic dose response to glycogen modulation:

"...one challenge is to titrate the threshold for muscle glycogen content that might enhance the metabolic adaptations without causing complications associated with fatigue or changes in the net protein balance." [79]

Applying Heat to Muscle:

- used for treating severe muscle injuries
- may improve recovery time

- leads to higher local blood flow => delivery of more oxygen and nutrients to the injury site => possible faster repair
- upregulates the activity of HSPs (heat shock proteins)

Similar to muscle glycogen modulation, Peake and colleagues (2015) report contrasting evidence here:

"Heat preconditioning also increases the activation of Akt, mTOR, ribosomal protein S6, and eukaryotic translation initiation factor 4E-binding protein 1 (EIF4E-BP1) after resistance exercise. In contrast with these studies, others have reported no benefits of heat preconditioning on the recovery of strength, range of motion, edema, or soreness after eccentric exercise." [79]

Antioxidant Supplementation:

According to Peake et al. (2015), there have only been a few studies to analyze protocols involving the combination of resistance training and antioxidant supplementation. And, to nobody's surprise, they report variable findings:

- in **two studies**: no improvement in muscle strength or performance with vitamins C and E supplementation
- in **another study**: vitamins C and E supplementation attenuates hypertrophy response

"Thus, some evidence supports blunting of the cell signaling pathways with antioxidant supplementation following resistance exercise, although the effects on functional outcomes remain equivocal." [79]

From their analysis of the current evidence, Peake and colleagues (2015) think that antioxidant supplementation (vit. C and E) may *"dampen exercise-induced hormesis — at least at the cellular level"*, but they cannot ascertain if these responses have an impact on long-term exercise performance [79].

Cryotherapy:

- **local ice application** - common treatment for soft injuries
- **cold water immersion (CWI)** - attenuates muscle adaptation to training, by currently unknown mechanisms.

Peake et al. (2015) hypothesize that this dampening effect could be because of lower muscle blood flow (from CWI), which translates to lower angiogenesis and lower protein synthesis [79].

- post-exercise **cryotherapy** - may reduce muscle soreness and minimize subsequent tissue damage. But, according to these researchers:

"...by attenuating some key inflammatory reactions (e.g., macrophage infiltration) in skeletal muscle, cryotherapy may also block the production and release of important growth factors and the activity of satellite cells, which are important mediators of muscle repair and adaptation." [79]

Thus, the possible short-term benefits of cryotherapy can be outweighed by possible long-term detrimental effects.

I suspect that the timing of all these interventions is a crucial factor that can make them more positive or negative for long-term health and strength benefits from exercise. A cryotherapy strategy that is implemented immediately after a workout session may be more detrimental than one applied a couple of hours post training.

Moreover, using heat stress immediately post work (higher blood flow => more nutrients delivered, higher HSP activity, etc) and cold stress after a couple of hours after workout (to assist recovery) may make more sense. A practical example:

- sauna immediately after RT session, CWI 5-6 hours post RT session.

Similarly, other protocols can be implemented strategically, in a combined way or in isolation, to potentiate the positive adaptive benefits of exercise. Now, let me briefly discuss the possible positive cognitive effects of exercise.

According to Gradari and colleagues (2016), exercise can increase the availability and the function of neurotransmitters like norepinephrine, glutamate, dopamine and serotonin [80].

In combination with dietary stress from food restriction, exercise induces mild metabolic stress on neural cells (higher intracellular Ca2+ and higher ROS). Then:

"This pathway activates several transcription factors like CREB and NF-kB, controlling BDNF and antiapoptotic gene (such as Bcl-2) expression. These factors drive cell survival, synaptic plasticity and neurogenesis processes." [80]

Exercise alone can increase neurogenesis in the hippocampus, while environmental enrichment can increase the survival of immature neurons [80]. Counter intuitively, when neural stem cells are treated with low level physical, pharmacological, and chemical stimuli (that would be toxic in higher doses), this intervention provides protection for cell precursors in conditions of neurodegenerative diseases [80].

Even though I have devoted extensive paper-space to the topic of stressors and adaptive responses in exercise physiology, there is still much to be explored.

Next, I will discuss stressors and adaptive responses in the contexts of nutrition, lack of nutrition, food psychopathologies, supplementation and other similar concepts.

Chapter 4:
Nutrition and Adaptive Stress Responses

Have you ever thought about food as being something more than just a means to stave off hunger? I'm sure you have. We all do. In fact, each and every one of us nurtures a personal relationship with food, admittedly or not. We all have our favorite dishes and desserts, which we enjoy consuming once, twice or multiple times a day. Some people, more than others, consider food as being a crucial factor to their health. This makes them more careful about their food selection; sometimes too careful.

Some people believe in the existence of super-foods, when there is no solid scientific rationale for their support. Some believe in curing diseases with food alone; some believe that over-consuming a nutrient or a supplement can lead to superior health benefits.

I think that we eat too much and too often, sometimes developing twisted rationalizations in support of certain dietary beliefs, and in the most extreme of cases our dietary habits can turn into food psychopathologies.

In this chapter I purpose to explore the rationale behind nutrition or its absence as being a positive stressor. While the supply of food alone can serve as a stressor to the body (caloric restriction, fasting, IF, etc), some food constituents can also inherently serve as stressors by triggering adaptive responses - a concept that you should be very familiar with by now). Dose-response relationships, timing, tolerance buildup, sensitization and desensitization will be discussed in this context.

I also want to touch upon more sensitive subjects that involve abnormal relationships with food and feeding. This is what I am going to discuss next.

Food Psychopathologies

The field of psychopathology explores mental disorders in an effort to understand their biologic, genetic, social, and psychological causes. Food psychopathologies are mental disorders that develop on the basis of an abnormal relationship with food and with eating habits.

Some researchers think of this as being yet another diagnosis fad of professionals wishing to invent new fields of study. But, is it? Let me get into a few articles and see if there really is a rationale behind these food driven disorders. I'll also try to see how this relates to the concept of stress.

In an article from 2011 published in *Eating Disorders,* Vandereycken wanted to determine whether 4 new eating disorders could be considered legitimate. The title of the article is self-explanatory: 'Media hype, diagnostic fad or genuine disorder?' [82]

One of these four disorders is **orthorexia nervosa**, a condition encountered in people who are so obsessed with healthy eating that their eating behavior can lead to malnutrition. The name of this disorder can make us think of anorexia nervosa, another psychopathology in which the subject is obsessively focused on weight loss; anorexia is characterized by the use of unhealthy methods for losing weight.

Another one of the four disorders is the **Night Eating Syndrome**, which has been around since the 1950s and has regained popularity with the discussion around binge eating disorders [82]. It involves evening hyperphagia (consuming 25% or more of the daily total calories after the evening meal) and waking up at night to consume food. While interesting, I will not discuss it in detail.

The remaining two eating disorders are **Muscle Dysmorphia** and **Emetophobia**.

In Muscle Dysmorphia, often referred to as Reverse Anorexia, subjects are obsessed with the idea of being too skinny or not muscular enough [82]. This condition is mostly prevalent in males. Being familiar with the 'gym' culture, I know that some 'bros' refer to this condition as bigorexia. A web search for photos about 'bigorexia' or 'muscle dysmorphia' may be revealing.

Emetophobia involves avoiding certain foods because of the fear of vomiting. I can relate this to a personal childhood experience: I remember that I used to lock myself into my room while my parents were cooking fish in the crock-pot. I could not stand its smell, and even the slightest of its scent would have me throw up instantly. It is not that I enjoy eating fish now, as an adult, but I am a bit more tolerant to its 'fishy' smell.

Out of these four, I'm going to expand the discussion on orthorexia nervosa because I suspect that many people deal with a certain form of it, milder or more severe. I've seen it in myself, and I now see it more often in social media circles (frequency bias?). Here is what I think:

Some of us obsess with the purity and 'organic'-ity of foods, always trying to consume non-GMO (a term that is so poorly understood by most people) and 'you-name-it'-free (gluten, BPA, chemical, etc), when these are, for the most part, marketing gimmicks tailored to the less science educated people.

Trying to consume only 'pure' foods (if that is even possible) means removing all dietary stress; it leaves little room for nutritionally challenging the body. An example from the other extreme is people who are prone to ingesting higher doses of arsenic because of the environment they live in. How do you think their bodies respond? They are generally healthy because

112

they have adapted to processing and removing arsenic better than those living in environments that leak less arsenic into water and food. I'll discuss this particular example later in the book.

I'm not saying that you should not be careful with what goes into your mouth. But if you take it to a level of obsession and you dedicate your life exclusively to food sourcing and prepping, this may do you no good. Not only that it is too time consuming, but that it is also socially isolating and it limits the spectrum of food one can eat. A sensible approach in this case, in my view, would be the implementation of The 80/20 Pareto Principle - be consistent 80% of the time, be less careful for the remaining 20%. Examples:

- eat whole foods - don't obsess about 'non-GMO' labels
- eat whole foods most of the time - allow yourself to indulge every once in while

More importantly, think of the unwanted psychologic stress you may induce to yourself when purposing for the unattainable and blurry concept of food purity. Here's an example:

The label says it's organic meat. But what if they fed grains to the chickens every now and then? What if the water consumed by the chickens contained some level of toxic chemicals? Can you see where I am going? There will always be a level of uncertainty that will dismiss purity.

These represent my quick views on the concept of orthorexia. But let's see some scientific literature on the subject.

Orthorexia was coined by Steven Bratman in 1996. It comes from the combination of two Greek terms [83]:

'orthos' - right

'orexis' - which resembles appetite (for food)

According to Bartrina (2007), orthorexia is an obsessive compulsive disorder, characterized by extreme care for food selection [84]:

"This ritual leads to a very restrictive diet and social isolation as a compensation. Orthorexics obsessively avoid foods which may contain artificial colours, flavours, preservant agents, pesticide residues or genetically modified ingredients, unhealthy fats, foods containing too much salt or too much sugar and other components. The way of preparation, kitchenware and other tools used are also part of the obsessive ritual." [84]

Bartrina (2007) thinks that the higher risk groups for developing orthorexia are women, adolescents and those who practice sports such as bodybuilding. I would also include celebrities, 'food junkies' and 'food purists' into this.

Is there any clinical basis for Orthorexia Nervosa? Koven and Abry (2015) decided to investigate this matter [85]. They wanted to identify the prevalence, known symptoms, neuro-profile and the treatment of orthorexia. In their words:

"Neuropsychological data suggest that orthorexic symptoms are independently associated with key facets of executive dysfunction." [85]

Executive dysfunction may translate into neurocortex pathology. While there is no precise therapeutic prescription for orthorexia (one reason being its novelty), *"current best practices suggest that orthorexia can successfully be treated with a combination of cognitive-behavioral therapy, psychoeducation, and medication."* [85]

In an earlier study, Donini and colleagues (2004), decided to measure the prevalence of Orthorexia Nervosa. They enrolled 404 subjects. Their diagnosing of orthorexia was based *"on both the presence of a disorder with obsessive-compulsive personality features and an exaggerated healthy eating behaviour pattern."* [86]

28 subjects were found to suffer from orthorexia (6.9% of 404). Researchers remarked that orthorexia is more prevalent in men and in people with lower levels of education. This is somewhat different from what the earlier study had found (women - higher category risk). It would be interesting to get a more precise view of the subjects in both of these studies.

Donini et al. (2004) report:

"The orthorexic subjects attribute characteristics that show their specific "feelings" towards food ("dangerous" to describe a conserved product, "artificial" for industrially produced products, "healthy" for biological produce) and demonstrate a strong or uncontrollable desire to eat when feeling nervous, excited, happy or guilty." [86]

My current view about this:

- orthorexic behavior => incompatible with normal life
- focus on food purity => removes the potential positive effects of dietary stressors
- the body is not challenged to eliminate unwanted chemicals
- paradoxically, it can debilitate body function.

Please take my view with the adequate amount of common-sense:

I'm not saying that one should sprinkle arsenic atop of their meals. I'm suggesting that 'impure' foods (whatever 'impure' means) may not be as detrimental as we think, if other aspects of one's life are given appropriate consideration (i.e. exercise, sleep, etc.).

Next, we'll explore the molecular mechanisms of food stressors and the body's adaptive responses to it.

Molecular Mechanisms of Dietary Stress

Out of the innumerable pathways and mechanisms that could be discussed in this context, I am only going to focus on a few that I consider more important. These molecular factors and pathways include: Nrf2, HSPs, NF-κB, SIRT1, and FOXO.

Nrf2

The cellular endogenous defense to oxidation agents is controlled by various pathways, one of which is regulated by Nrf2, which is a transcription factor. Nrf2 regulates the transcription of more than 500 genes, most of which are involved in cytoprotection.

Under normal conditions, Nrf2 is sequestered/bound to Keap1 in the cytoplasm. Under conditions of oxidative or chemical stress (either exogenous or endogenous), Nrf2 evades Keap1, accumulates inside the nucleus and leads to the activation of different genes.

According to Pall and Levine (2015) [87]:

"Nrf2 produces cytoprotection by detoxification mechanisms leading to increased detoxification and excretion of both organic xenobiotics and toxic metals; its action via over two dozen genes increases highly coordinated antioxidant activities; it produces major anti-inflammatory changes; it stimulates mitochondrial biogenesis and otherwise improves mitochondrial function; and it stimulates autophagy, removing toxic protein aggregates and dysfunctional organelles."

Some of the endogenous activators of Nrf2 include: hypochlorous acid, hydrogen peroxide, peroxynitrite,

116

isoprostanes, and others. Similarly, there are numerous exogenous agents and environmental factors known to activate Nrf2. Some examples are: heavy metals, quinones, selenium compounds, polyphenols, phenolic acids, carotenoids, chalcones and isothiocyanates. Other factors that are known to raise Nrf2 activity are calorie restriction, exercise, and low level oxidative stress. I would assume that fasting can be included in this list as well.

According to Suresh and Le Bourg (2014) [51]:

"Regardless of the designation, it is evident that the intake of Nrf2-inducing substances as part of the daily diet, directly or indirectly, generates mild electrophilic stress that enhances the cellular capacity to cope with exogenous stressors and improves their resistance against oxidizing environmental stimuli." [51]

Higher Nrf2 levels may be preferable as they could potentially prevent or treat conditions like cardiovascular disease, toxic liver damage, kidney disease, metabolic disorders, inflammatory bowel disease, and others [87].

The average person, today, is exposed to high levels of cellular perturbing agents so it would make sense to desire for increased Nrf2 activity which can promote cytoprotection. According to Pall and Levine (2015) [87]:

"The two most healthful diets known, the traditional Mediterranean and Okinawan diets, and the Paleolithic diet are all thought to be rich in Nrf2 raising nutrients, whereas modern diets are deficient in such nutrients." [87]

Here is an overall picture of the Nrf2 regulatory system:

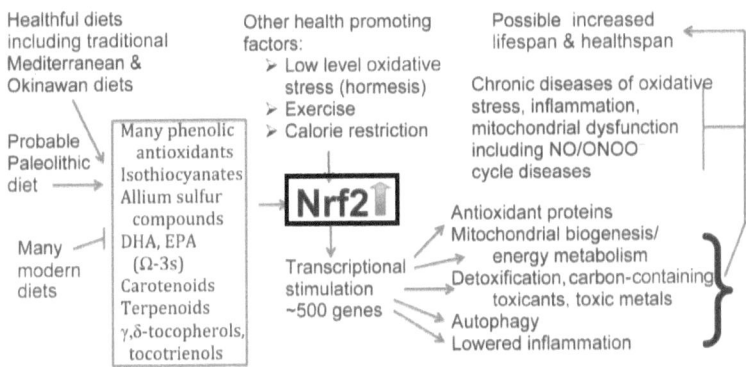

Adapted from Pall and Levine (2015) [87]

Even though higher Nrf2 levels are overall preferable, chronic elevation of Nrf2 may not be beneficial, as it may produce undesired pathophysiological effects.

Instead of focusing on the minute details of optimizing Nrf2 activity (which, at the moment, may not be quantifiable and approachable - being more like a guess work), I'd suggest looking at the overall picture. Numerous dietary factors, that have been mentioned and that I will mention in subsequent sections, act via numerous pathways (including Nrf2). Experimenting with, adjusting them, and observing what works for one's better health is something that I would pursue.

To be more clear: a health goal should not consist of better Nrf2 activation because you cannot conveniently measure its levels. Plus, you do not know its exact interactions with other pathways and their interdependent health effects. Instead, use dietary stressors to make more convenient and quantifiable subjective (how you feel) and objective observations (bodyweight progression, blood biomarkers, body composition, etc).

HSPs

Heat shock proteins have been introduced previously in the book. These proteins are expressed in all cell types, especially in conditions of temperature stress and/or other stresses (including dietary stress), directly or indirectly [51].

NF-κB

Nuclear factor κB is a transcription factor that can be activated by parasites, bacteria, viruses, radiation, ROS and other insults. According to Suresh and Le Bourg (2014) [51]:

"One of the first physiologically essential functions of NF-κB has been unraveled in the development of the immune system."

Involved in the cellular response to harmful stimuli, the activation of this factor can promote different responses: inflammatory response, immune response, cell proliferation response, and cell survival are to name a few. If endogenous signals cannot terminate NF-κB activation appropriately, the cell will die.

There are several endogenous and exogenous inhibitors of NF-κB. One of the mechanisms of inhibition is through the inhibition of PARP-1 (enzyme):

"In a screening of a broad range of dietary flavonoids, we identified among others myricetin, tricetin, quercetin, and fisetin, as well as theophylline and caffeine metabolites, as significant PARP-1 inhibitors in vitro." [51]

I have conflicting feelings regarding the efficiency and appropriateness of trying to control such delicate cellular mechanisms, outside of the context of a severe condition.

SIRT1

Another molecular factor in the cellular response to different stressors is SIRT1. Conditions of low energy, such as calorie restriction and fasting, lead to the activation of SIRT1, while high-energy states, such as the fed state, promote its inactivation. There are several positive outcomes associated with the activation of SIRT1, and I will get into them in an upcoming section.

FOXO

There are multiple transcription factors included in the FOXO family and their effects (when active) have been observed in the signaling pathways of apoptosis, stress resistance, cell proliferation and atrophy. Activation of FOXO can have positive effects on tolerance to stressors, as well as lifespan:

"Excitingly, a few recently published preliminary reports show that some polyphenols, such as EGCG, the major polyphenol in green tea; baicalein, a trihydroxyflavone; and resveratrol, can modulate FOXO activity in mammalian cells." [51]

Nutritional Components to Activate Cell Stress Responses

The pathways that I mentioned earlier have been shown to induce beneficial effects in the adaptive response of cells to stressors. There are nutritional components that can activate one or more of these pathways at the same time. Consumption of phytochemicals, for example, is known to have a biphasic dose-response, with positive effects at low doses and possible negative effects at higher doses.

While it has been known for a while that supplementing with antioxidants may not confer positive health effects (sometimes it can even be detrimental), the same thing cannot be said of the antioxidants that come in foods.

Both plant antioxidants and phytochemicals remain controversial because (as far as I know) there is no solid evidence of their efficacy. Along the same lines:

"Another matter is represented by the relative lack of potency and the consequent large doses needed to be employed to reach the biological effect. One possible solution for these problems is to modify the structure of lead hormetic phytochemicals, by using medicinal chemistry, to develop new compounds exhibiting selectivity for only one target and increased potency." [88]

Until (and if) this type of research receives more attention, we should pay a closer look at the plant compounds for which there is evidence (good or bad) that they act as stressors (at low doses). Some effects include increased glutathione levels and higher activity of enzymes such as superoxide dismutase, thioredoxin reductase and glutathione peroxidase - thus, marking and overall increased cellular antioxidative activity.

According to Birringer (2011) [89], some of these compounds are:

- allicin from garlic
- lipoic acid - as in spinach and broccoli
- sulphoraphane - as in cauliflower, broccoli and kale:

"Sulforaphane is a phytochemical present in high amounts in broccoli sprouts and cruciferous vegetables. It is known to activate the Nrf2-ARE stress response pathway in a variety of cells including neurons." [91]

- isothiocyanates - as in cabbage, watercress, and mustard
- crocetin
- phytanic acid and pristanic acid

- palmitic and linoleic acid
- falcarinol and falcarindiol - as in carrots and celery
- quercetin
- resveratrol - as in grapes, blueberries, and red wine
- carnosic acid - as in Rosemary

Hooper and colleagues (2010) [90] add a few more to this list:

- salicylate - as in cucumbers
- curcumin - as in curcuma
- carvacrol - as in oregano
- ascorbic acid
- abscisic acid
- catechins and epicatechins - as in green tea
- and a few others.

According to Son, Camandola and Mattson (2008) [91], some of these phytochemicals enhance detoxification pathways:

"Potentially noxious chemicals ingested with food undergo enzymatic metabolism in a coordinated process involving phase I, II and III enzymes; metabolites are then excreted from the body. Some such phytochemicals induce the expression of phase II enzymes via the Nrf2/ARE pathway." [91]

Another known theory in the circle of researchers interested in toxicology and the biology of adaptation is the xenohormesis theory. With its sophisticated and unintelligible name, you can easily guess that I'm not particularly convinced by its proponents, but I think it deserves further attention and testing within the scientific community.

According to the xenohormesis theory, stressed plants produce compounds that can enhance not only their own stress resistance but also that of the organisms that consume them. From Hooper and colleagues (2010) [90]:

"A prime example of such an unexpected outcome is observed in the production of wine, where the best grapes in terms of taste and health benefit often result from relatively dry, sun-exposed, infertile soil."

Researchers explain that resveratrol (from red wine) synthesis is stimulated by ozone, exposure to UV light and other pathogens and its effect is to confer protection to the plant from these insults. Resveratrol is also known to activate the mammalian stress response in different model organisms, leading to a cascade of positive health and longevity benefits.

Examples of similar xenohormetic compounds are: curcumin, sulphoraphane, and green tea catechins and epicatechins:

"These compounds modulate key pathways that control inflammation, the energy status of cells, and cellular stress responses in a way that is predicted to increase health and survival of the organism." [92]

Here is how the story goes, according to Morris (2008):

"Under stressful conditions such as cold or drought, when plants ramp up their production of these specialized chemical compounds, by eating the plants, the benefit is transferred to animals." [93]

Do I think of this theory as being a 'bit' over-confabulated? Yes. But I also think it needs more scrutiny, because if it turns out to be a widely encountered mechanism - common in plants and animals - we could benefit from its practical implications and applications.

Aside of these phytochemicals and plant compounds, alcohol has, in some studies, been shown to elicit similar dose-response effects:

"Although resveratrol has attained notoriety for its health benefits, alcohol itself, at low doses, can confer benefits by lowering cardiovascular risk. The relationship between consumption of ethanol, from any alcoholic beverage, and cardiovascular risk is J-shaped. Moderate intake is associated with a lower risk than no or a higher intake." [93]

Do not get too excited though, because these effects may not be present in healthy people; thus it would make no sense for alcohol consumption. I suspect that low-to-moderate, infrequent consumption, in healthy people, may not be detrimental to health. Notice that I am not saying that it can be helpful either. Alcohol is a stressor that your body can deal with (every now and then), if it does not have too many other stressors to attend to.

I have to caution that with frequent/chronic use, according to the World Health Organization (2015):

"The harmful use of alcohol results in the death of 3.3 million people annually. There are 60 different types of diseases where alcohol has a significant causal role. It also causes harm to the well-being and health of people around the drinker." [94]

An appropriate take home message from this section would be to increase and diversify your consumption of vegetables and other plant foods rich in polyphenols, phytochemicals and similar compounds. As per Morris (2008):

"The various flavonoids have, moreover, additive and synergistic effects. Therefore an intake of a combination of flavonoids is most likely going to be preferable to ingestion of one or a few, and consumption of natural sources to get these would appear desirable." [93]

In the next section I will keep my focus on the nutritional aspect of positive physiologic stress, but I will discuss two of its different facets: calorie restriction and fasting (intermittent and/or prolonged).

Physiologic Stress from Energy Supply Manipulation

I'll start 'lightly' and opinionated...

Most of us assume that food availability has been the same throughout human history. We seldom question the rationale of consuming 3 or more meals a day plus snacks. This type of meal partitioning has probably grown into the norm due to its societal convenience: eat before work, eat sometime mid-day, eat at night with the family; have some bits of food in-between.

Not only society, but also blood sugar fluctuations can drive this type of eating regimen - assuming that one consumes a regular diet - not devoid of carbohydrates. I think that much of the nutrition science literature is built on this type of feeding cycle, while less than decent research is conducted on feeding protocols that are different, non-regular and asynchronous.

There is much less good research, to my knowledge, on irregular eating, on caloric deprivation and restriction and on fasting, compared to the norm - regular eating. Please do not get me wrong: there is literature on this topic, but a lot of it is blurry, inconclusive, and often, statistically flawed.

Some researchers point, based on cited evidence, that we are not evolved to consume so much food everyday. Regulatory agencies have created daily caloric recommendations based on an observed ability to maintain (bodyweight) homeostasis in certain populations. Thus, to maintain weight: active, healthy, adult males should consume around 2,500 kcals per day, while active, healthy, adult females should purpose for ~2,000 kcals.

There is nothing wrong in taking such a recommendation as a starting point. The individual however, should assess an approximate required daily caloric intake based on the numerous variables in their life, taking into consideration the dynamic nature of energy requirements. Additionally, there are other feeding/non-feeding regimens different from the '3 meals/day' that are worth exploring for health betterment and maintenance. Here I will focus on calorie restriction, periodic and intermittent fasting - though there are many more 'out there'.

I will begin with the assumption that throughout our history we may not have had the same availability to food that we have today. Even though this may make sense, we do not really know the exact details/intricacies of how people lived their lives in the past; we make a lot of assumptions.

According to Martin and colleagues (2010) [95]:

"The ability to adapt to varying levels of available energy in the form of food in the environment has allowed species to propagate and also thrive during times of energy surplus. However, in times when there is scant food available, similar evolutionary pressures have ensured that physiological systems can adapt to and utilize this food scarcity to their advantage."

The mechanisms of adaptive homeostasis may allow humans to function on a variety of energy intake protocols. I think that is one of the reasons we have successfully inhabited a diversified range of our planet's environments. In times of plenty we build our bodies and store for times of scarcity. In times of scarcity we make our bodies more resilient; the simple logic...

The problem of today is that there is not much room left for times of scarcity. We are in the 'plenty' mode continuously, never stressing our bodies with 'scarcity'.

According to Martin, Mattson, and Maudsley (2006) [96], both whole body and cellular physiology are impacted by caloric restriction and fasting. Researchers think that the main beneficial stressor of calorie restriction is the attenuated production of energy [95].

In terms of whole body physiology, they enumerate the following benefits of dietary restriction [96]:

- neuroprotection, in the central nervous system
- better circulation through: improved glycemia, lower IIS, higher cortisol (it can be good in some situations), activity of trophic factors like BDNF, and ketogenesis
- higher hepatic stress protection
- increased tolerance to stress (a vague and unspecific effect).

In terms of cellular physiology, they enumerate the following benefits of calorie restriction and fasting [96]:

- better energy metabolism: higher insulin sensitivity, higher fat mobilization and increased PPAR activation
- higher activity of heat shock proteins => protein stability
- higher activity of sirtuins => DNA stability
- better cell survival through the upregulation of FoxO and BDNF:

"During these times of energy deficit, cell survival is supported by the activation of forkhead box-other (FoxO) transcription factors and through the generation of neurotrophic agents such as brain-derived neurotrophic factor (BDNF)." [96]

Members of the FOXO protein family are responsible with the translation of environmental stimuli (such as stress induce by dietary restriction) into potentially beneficial patterns of gene expression [96].

Martin and colleagues (2010) think that calorie restriction induced production of ketones may not only provide alternative sources of energy in the context of lower circulating glucose but can also elicit potent cytoprotective effects [95].

Because calorie restriction is not appealing to many people, there is some research that promotes the use of so called 'calorie restriction mimetics'. I am personally not excited about using this type of intervention as a primary mean to improve health but, nevertheless, I will mention these mimetics and their supposed mechanisms of action. This book is about appropriate stress exposure and its potential positive adaptive nature, and not about stress-avoidance. That is why I am in favor of calorie restriction and some forms of fasting as primary strategies for benefiting from dietary stress and, if there's some 'room' left, CR mimetics could be used optionally.

Testa and colleagues (2014) [98] name a few agents that mimic the calorie-restricted state: rapamycin, 2-deoxiglucose, resveratrol, lipoic acid, metformin and some compounds from the thiazolidinediones family. The molecular targets of these mimetics include: SIRT1, AMPk, TOR, and FoxO. Most CR mimetics act on more than one of these pathways and they often act interdependently:

"SIRT-1, known to modulate the activity of many proteins associated with energy metabolism, stress resistance, cell survival and longevity, including FoxO and PGC-1, is activated by 2-DG, resveratrol and the thiazolidinediones. These latter two agents, together with metformin, activate AMPK, which in turn inhibits TOR." [98]

Another strategy of energy restriction is fasting. It can take many forms based on its duration and the amount of energy intake that is restricted. An easier strategy of fasting is daily intermittent fasting, while a more advanced one involves prolonged water fasting. In-between are countless of variations.

As pointed by Lam and Ravussin (2014), fasting can provide protection to damage from oxidation by upregulating the expression of proteins and pathways involved in stress response. By using endogenous fat (adipose tissue) as an energy substrate and by upregulating beta-oxidation, fewer reactive oxygen species should be generated because of bypassing complex I in the electron transport chain (this is mostly theoretical) [97].

When people fast and feast, such as in the case of daily intermittent fasting, common sense would imply that the periods of dietary energy deprivation should be compensated by spontaneous increase in calories during feasting, in order to maintain homeostasis. More simply put, if people fast for 20 hours every day, they should be able to consume all their required calories (for dietary homeostasis) in the remaining 4-hour feeding window. But this is not the case, as referenced by Lam and Ravussin (2014) in a series of human experiments [97]:

- 3 weeks of alternate day fasting => significant weight loss in non-obese healthy subjects
- 8 weeks of alternate day modified fasting (ADMF) in obese: ad lib. intake during feast days, 25% of DER (daily energy requirement) during fast days => overall 37% caloric restriction and ~5.6kg average weight loss
- 6 months of ADMF in overweight women: 25% of DER 2 days/week, ad lib. intake (eat as much as they wanted) for 5 days/week => overall ~30% reduction in energy intake [97]

These studies suggest that there is an unintentional reduction in total energy intake with such feeding strategies. I think that these may be more approachable and appealing to some people who want to lose weight, compared to focusing on caloric restriction alone (with multiple meals/day evenly distributed).

I would be careful in analyzing and extrapolating conclusions from studies in overweight and obese people, as they may lead to different outcomes that in normal weight people. Nevertheless, I am glad that we have some research literature in humans on this topic, which provides us with some knowledge on the effects of different feeding/fasting protocols.

Some of the possible positive mechanisms of fasting, as pointed out by Lam and Ravussin (2014) [97] are:

- higher mitochondrial metabolism during fasting and during feeding => cyclic higher ROS production => stimulation of endogenous anti-oxidative systems
- fasting stimulates HPA axis => production of glucocorticoids.

Moreover:

"Intermittent flux of energy substrates and the alternating catabolism and anabolism increase the expression and probably the activity of sirtuin 1 (SIRT1), which improves cellular defense, energy metabolism, and cognition function. Together with its effect on reducing oxidative molecular damage, SIRT1 positively influences metabolic, physical and functional health, and therefore increases lifespan and healthspan." [97]

These authors remark that adherence to fasting may be more achievable compared to a regimen of chronic caloric restriction, but they could not foresee how people would adapt to food restriction every other day [97]. I am inclined to say that it may be easier to follow a daily intermittent fasting strategy for this purpose, regardless of its design: intermittent fasting of 16:8, 18:6, 20:4, 22:2, and so on.

Both calorie restriction and fasting (IF and PF - with all their 'flavors') represent perturbations of homeostasis, unlike a feeding protocol characterized by several meals a day, everyday. I think they represent positive dietary stressors with health benefits resulting from the adaptive molecular and whole-body responses. The main reason I did not go into extensive detail with respect to these dietary strategies is because I have touched upon them at length in my previous books.

In the past, I may have held a more rigid and inflexible opinion regarding caloric restriction and fasting. My personal experimentation outside of such fixated strategies, as well as my literature research on these topics expanded my vision and I may, now, possess a more flexible view. Additionally, I am opened to new theories, especially if it involves practical experimentation on the side; the stress-response perspective of these topics is much of my current interest.

A few concepts that are worth further pursuit, in light of positive stress and stressors may include: microbiota and the gut-brain axis, immunology and immune system modulation, as well as exploiting stressors and stress response relationships for disease management. These may be the subject of another book. Who knows?

Introducing and exploring adaptive stress response is the major theme of this book. So far, we have looked into exercise stress and dietary stress because I think they are of greater importance. In the remainder of the book, I will discuss other, more unexplored and controversial (to be read 'blurry') topics involving adaptive stress: cold and heat stress, toxicology and stress from radiation, cognitive stress (touch at length in other books - but not necessarily from a physiologic perspective), and aging. I will conclude with a theoretical and personal view of stress in light on the 'anti-fragility' concept, derived from the great essays of Nicholas Nassim Taleb. Proceed, shall we?

Chapter 5:
Temperature Stress

Comfort and security make it easier for us to enjoy the great things in life, but they are not, in themselves, great and enjoyable aims.

Hans Selye

Earlier in the book, I described the concepts of homeostasis and adaptive homeostasis referring to the tendency of the human body to maintain a state of equilibrium/normalcy. One of the main homeostatic processes is the preservation of constant body temperature of approximately 37°C. Cellular and molecular adaptive systems work for the purpose of maintaining such thermal homeostasis.

Perturbations in body temperature cause stress. Such perturbations can come from localized/systemic inflammation causing an increase in temperature or from deliberate/non-deliberate exposure to higher or lower temperature; it could come from various other causes too. The system usually responds adaptively.

In case of thermal stress from heat or cold exposure, the main purpose of the response is to restore normal temperature. 'Side' effects may imply better resistance of the cells/system to future perturbations from the same stressor. When thermal stress involves inflammation as a result of a disease/disorder state (infection, bone rupture, etc), the system's response is, at least, dual in nature - fight the disordered state, return normal temperature, if not much more complex.

Hot and Freezing, far from Normal

Here I am going to focus on temperature stress as a result of deliberate heat or cold exposure. Examples of stressors can be hyperthermic, hypothermic and a more extreme form can come from cryotherapy.

According to Scapagnini et al. (2014) [99]:

"...mild heat relates to the capacity of living systems to respond to stress, and accumulating evidences show that transfer of thermal energy into or out of the body causes physiological changes because of molecular or cellular responses to adaptation."

In case of hyperthermic stress, the main molecular response involves the upregulation of heat shock proteins. As I discussed in chapter 2, HSPs are stress proteins involved in body's response to heat shock; they stimulate proteolysis, they prevent protein degradation, and they also act in protein refolding and protein remodeling. Better described by Scapagnini and colleagues (2014):

"HSPs are highly conserved and ubiquitous molecular chaperones with multifunctional roles to prevent proteotoxic stress–induced denaturation of other proteins through holding and folding pathways." [99]

The mechanisms, as explored in different organisms, are thought to be:

1. Stressors activate heat shock factors (HSFs)
2. They separate from HSPs and get phosphorylated
3. They enter the nucleus and attach to HSEs (heat shock elements)
4. They lead to the creation of new HSPs, which can further aid in the adaptive cellular response.

There are a few strategies one can implement to induce a positive adaptive response from mild heat stress. The cheapest and, in my view, probably the most readily implementable stressor of this kind is physical exercise. Others include the use of saunas, as well as the ingestion of different plant extracts - think of capsaicin, as in chili pepper.

While heat saunas are extensively acclaimed to elicit numerous health benefits, I have yet to find good studies to show clear and strong effects with respect to their efficacy in healthy humans. I do not want to demise their use however. Some proponents claim that they may help with issues of hypertension, post infarction care, and congestive heart failure [99]:

"One of the molecular mechanisms by which repeated sauna therapy improves endothelial function is the induction of endothelial nitric oxide synthase, as demonstrated in hamsters exposed to a far-infrared ray dry sauna system (39°C for 15 minutes) for 4 weeks. Repeated sauna therapy performed in patients at risk for lifestyle-related diseases has been found to significantly improve vascular endothelial function and to reduce both body weight and fasting plasma glucose." [99]

Other, more appealing (to me), protocols suggest using cold exposure prior to sauna. According to Scapagnini et al. (2014):

"The body reacts defensively against the reduced temperature by increasing many of its metabolic functions. Conversely, increased blood flow and muscle tone occur when the cold stress is over. An adaptation to repeated hot and cold stress may be involved in increased tolerance to stress and diseases. It was shown that the neuroendocrine and immune systems are challenged after thermal stress." [99]

I have used this type of protocol for a few months during the winter of 2015. I would take an extended (10-12 min) very cold shower. Immediately after, I would head to the gym and lift weights for 30 minutes to 1 hour. Then, I would go into the IR (infrared) sauna for 5 minutes, followed by another very cold shower. Sometimes I would skip the cold shower at home, while some other times I would take a warm shower after the IR sauna.

My focus was on the contrast of temperatures that I would expose myself to within a short timeframe. I cannot and will not claim for other than subjective positive measures of wellbeing as a result of what I did. I am looking forward to repeat and modify these experiments in the upcoming winters. I would advise against this type of experimentation, unless one is able to tolerate such extremes of temperature safely - without getting yourself harmed or killed during the process (to be read: Do not try this at home!). Let us now turn the attention to cold temperature stress.

Even though evidence seems to point out that humans may have evolved in moderate climates, we have the ability to tolerate and live within a large spectrum of Earth's climates. Age, body composition, gender, exercise, as well as the ability to adapt, all influence and may differentiate our ability to thermoregulate [100]. In an article published in the journal of *Aviation, space and environmental medicine* in 2004, researchers note:

"...cold stress can rapidly overwhelm the human thermoregulatory system, and the sudden fall in skin temperature associated with cold-water immersion can elicit the extremely hazardous "cold shock" responses." [100]

When exposure goes on for too long, the body may become impaired in its ability to thermoregulate and the risks of developing hypothermia and, eventually death, increase exponentially. The arms and the head account for sites of major heat loss [100, 101].

Two of the major mechanisms that compensate for heat loss are non-shivering and shivering thermogenesis. Both elevate the basal metabolic rate (BMR) of the organism - the amount of energy that is 'burned' over a certain period of time. In lower mammals, shivering thermogenesis can increase BMR for up to 3 times, while in higher mammals and in man, it can increase BMR for up to 5 times [100, 101].

135

I am very 'experienced' with deliberately putting myself into shivering thermogenesis. I have to admit that it is extremely unpleasant, very unpractical and very inconvenient. Cold and ice water immersion are two 'efficient' strategies for this purpose.

Important to note is that unlike cold-air exposure, we cannot remain for too long immersed in cold water, without going into excessive cooling:

"This is a result of the physical properties of water. The thermal conductivity of water is about 25 times greater and the volumetric specific heat of water under normal conditions is about 4,000 times greater than the respective values of air." [101]

Hence, we may have trouble thermoregulating even in water at relatively moderate temperatures of 20 - 25°C. Still, I think that temperature stress from cold water immersion can be used to increase body's stress resistance, which is one of the reasons I have used it for so long. Modulating the dose to lower levels and time-restricting the exposure are key to eliciting benefits from cold stress; optimizing for intensity (the feeling that you are 'miserably' cold) is important too.

Shivering thermogenesis leads to heat production by involuntary muscle contractions; the process takes energy from the hydrolysis of ATP to ADP and Pi (hence, the increase in BMR). As described in a technical memorandum for NASA's Ames Research Center in 1989:

"The rapid formation of ADP during shivering accelerates substrate oxidation in mitochondria, which is accompanied by a loss of energy as heat. Although carbohydrates are the important fuel for contracting muscle there is no longer any doubt that oxidation of fat plays a vital role in providing energy for sustained shivering." [101]

Shivering leads to higher uptake of glucose in the muscles, even though cold exposure inhibits the secretion of insulin to a large extent, but not completely; as a result, more fatty acids are mobilized for energy utilization. Kaciub-Uscilko and Greenleaf (1989) point out that fasted animals fail to upregulate the uptake of glucose in muscles because muscles receive an enhanced supply of fatty acids and ketones:

"The enhanced lipolysis with concomitant release of free fatty acids and glycerol from adipose tissue to blood results from the cold-induced activation of the sympatho-adrenal system and reduced insulin secretion." [101]

Shivering muscles use only a part of the fatty acids derived from lipolysis, while the rest are repackaged in the liver and released back into circulation via VLDL, which can also be used by the muscles. Thyroid hormones T4 and T3 need to be present, so that upregulated lipolysis and thermogenesis can occur in cold exposure [101]. In the past, it was thought that neither the blood concentration of thyroid hormones nor their rate of turnover are affected by cold, but more recent studies have found that long-term cold exposure in humans leads to an accelerated elimination of T3, hence lower blood levels of T3 [102].

The metabolic mechanisms surrounding the responses to cold stress are even more complex if we consider the involvement of brown adipose tissue, which has been considered, for a long time, to be exclusive to neonates. More recently, it was discovered in adults too:

"During cold exposures the sympathetic nerve system is activated and noradrenaline is released to blood circulation and to BAT, where it leads to production of cAMP, lipolysis and free fatty acids. Free fatty acids open the mitochondrial proton channel protein in BAT. Protons enter the mitochondria and inhibit ATP synthesis (uncoupling)." [102]

While I remain to explore cold exposure at length in another book, I want to discuss a couple of research studies and personal experiments that are pertinent to cold stress.

Studies and Personal Experiments

Aside of the supposed benefits associated with thermogenesis, cold exposure has been thought to help with modulating the activation of the immune system, pain alleviation, and the potential activation of the vagus nerve; in shivering thermogenesis, these effects may be accentuated.

As I previously pointed out, I've experimented with cold exposure (cold showers) immediately after weight lifting. But is this a good thing to do?

First of all, I can 'safely' say it is not safe. Whether it is good or not remains a question to be put into context. Some studies point out that cold exposure immediately after working out may interfere with the positive pro-inflammatory effects of exercise.

The critical time frame when you may not want to interfere is about 1 hour.

As I often say, if you want to do a literature review on a certain hypothesis, there's at least one study conducted to support any argument you may have. What's more sad is that we often use this strategy when trying to prove our points, without even being aware of it and of the additional flaws a study may have. To read research and to understand what you are reading, you require a certain level of 'technical' knowledge on the subject. To be able to critically interpret it, you need very good skills in statistics, math and also knowledge of the inherent flaws of the human psyche.

Leaving this aside, I will look at some studies for post workout cold exposure and see if I can get something good out of them.

In one study, Ostrowski and colleagues (1999) wanted to know to what extent and by which time course vigorous exercise affects circulating inflammatory cytokines, cytokine inhibitors and anti-inflammatory cytokines [103]. Ten male subjects entered the study; they completed a marathon with an average of 3 hours and 26 minutes. Researchers took blood samples before, immediately after, and every 30 minutes for the following 4 hours (after the end of the prolonged exercise). Here's what they found:

- a 128-fold increase in IL-6, immediately after the race (vs. normal pre-exercise levels)
- a 39-fold increase in IL-1ra at one hour after race (vs. pre-exercise levels)
- a 27-fold increase in IL-10, immediately after race
- highest levels of IL1-beta, sTNF-r1, STNF-r2, TNF-α in the first hour after exercise

My main take-away message from this is that there is an increased pro-inflammatory (TNF-α and IL-6) response following strenuous exercise (endurance, in this case), which is balanced by higher activity of cytokine inhibitors and anti-inflammatory cytokines (sTNFs, IL-1ra, IL-10). This begs the question: how does cold exposure interfere with this response?

In one extensive report on cold stress, Dr. Patrick (2016) argues that from the studies she analyzed, she thinks that the first one hour after strength training represents an anabolic window and that trainees should be careful with their timing of cold exposure in this timeframe [104]; this was for strength, not endurance, training though.

As of now, I do not have a definitive/clear/strong opinion about this, especially because I experimented with immediate post-workout cold exposure without (subjectively) experiencing negative effects. Nevertheless, I think that it makes sense to be aware of the positive exercise induced inflammatory response, which could be impaired by immediate cold exposure. Context is, once again, of big importance: one may be more liberate in using immediate post workout cold exposure after endurance training versus strength training.

Another aspect to keep in mind is timing. If one engages in intensive strength training with the purpose of anabolism and they think that immediate post-work cold exposure may be detrimental to them, they could time the exposure to a later time of the day (i.e. 6-8 hours after training) or to non-workout days. I would apply the same rationale to the use of antioxidant and anti-inflammatory agents (think of supplements).

Other than for exercise related purposes, cold exposure may be of benefit in modulating the immune system or alleviating pain.

In a 12-week study of winter swimming versus cryotherapy, researchers recruited a group of 20 healthy female subjects and divided them into two groups: one group engaged in swimming in water that was between 0-2°C for 20 seconds 3 times/week, the other group engaged in whole body cryotherapy (exposure to -110°C) for two minutes 3 times/week. They took blood samples in weeks 1, 2, 4, 8 and 12 in days of non-exposure (to serve as control) and in days of exposure (cold specimens) at minute 0, 5 and 35 after exposure [105].

They found that plasma ACTH and cortisol in weeks 4 - 12 at 35 minutes after exposure were significantly lower compared to week 1. They thought that this could be attributed to habituation and that neither strategies (swimming and cryotherapy) stimulated the pituitary-adrenal-cortex axis [105].

Interestingly, I found the same argument in a few other studies. Circulating epinephrine did not change with either of the strategies, while norepinephrine was 2-3 folds higher for 12 weeks after cold exposure. In this study, IL1-beta, IL-6, and TNF-α were not affected by cold exposure. I have to add (even though it may be obvious) that subjects were not engaging in vigorous exercise.

In a different study from 2012, researchers studied 30 young healthy men (BMI 22 - 33) to determine if cryotherapy could be a viable strategy to improve their antioxidant capacity. Subjects were exposed, for 3 minutes, to very cold temperatures (-130°C) for 20 consecutive days. Researchers took blood samples before, 30 minutes after and then the following morning after exposure on days 1, 10, and 20. They reported a connection between exposure to very cold temperature and changes in the peroxidant and antioxidant status of the subjects [106]. According to Lubkowska et al. (2012):

"These changes seem to depend on the number of cryostimulations. After 20 daily treatments there was an increase in SOD, SOD:CAT ratio, a decrease in the concentration of reduced and oxidized glutathione and in the activity of GPx." [106]

It appears that cryotherapy increased the production of reactive oxygen species (ROS). This response was accompanied by compensatory adaptive changes:

"SOD activities appear sufficiently high and relatively uniform across tissues, suggesting that the removal of superoxide anion may not be a rate-limiting step. In comparison, GPx destroys the end products of the ROS generation pathway and its activity is relatively low. Increased glutathione reductase activity in subjects with normal BMI and absence of this reaction in people with elevated BMI may suggest the influence of

a factor released from adipose tissue that inhibits enzyme activity or synthesis. It is worth noting that these differences become clear only after the continuation of 20 WBC treatments." [106]

Superoxide dismutases (SOD) are the major antioxidants against superoxide radical (ROS), catalyzing it into molecular oxygen or hydrogen peroxide [107]. Glutathione reductase is a similar important enzyme.

Another interesting finding from this study involves uric acid. Ten cryotherapy sessions decreased uric acid secretion, which significantly increased after the series of 20 sessions, accompanied by a decrease in circulating albumin and ceruloplasmin. As per the researchers:

"It seems that the oxidant species produced during the first stage of WBC treatment (confirmed by a significant increase in 8-Iso-P) induces uric acid consumption. The results of the presented studies indicate a significant role of uric acid as a principal antioxidant molecule in the human body." [106]

I have personally experimented with the cryosauna, which is a form of cryotherapy. I entered the cold sauna, where I was exposed to a mix of vaporized liquid nitrogen and fresh air; the temperature was reduced to very low values, as low as -180°C or even lower. The duration of exposure is usually limited to 2-3 minutes, to prevent tissue damage.

In such a setting, the skin temperature drops to 0°C or lower, while core temperature remains unchanged (even minute drops in core temperature can be life-threatening); hence, skin cold receptors are activated, triggering a cascade of adaptive responses.

I only used the cryosauna once, in the fall of 2014, for the sake of experimentation. The experience was positive, it lead to immediate shivering thermogenesis, which lasted for a couple of hours. However, I do not think that this can be used conveniently because it is quite expensive. A 2 - 3 minute session in Romania costs ~$20, while in the U.S. it is approximately 5 times as much. There is a lot of marketing hype surrounding the use of cryosaunas. Many studies that are conducted within the field come from entities with a certain degree of 'skin in the game'; and this makes me skeptical...

Plus, cryosaunas are not as 'extremist' as they may appear. Exposure to cold air, even if it is at -180°C, is much more tolerable than spending 10 minutes in a cold bath or 5 minutes in an ice bath (remember air versus water conductivity from earlier in this chapter). I am not the only one to report this:

"Tolerance of cold in the cryogenic chamber with very low humidity is higher than during immersion in cold water, which may have a temperature of about 4°C during the winter season." [106]

Here is a photo from my cryosauna experience:

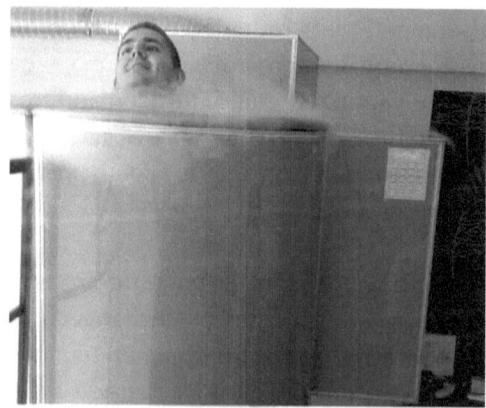

Cryosauna. Fall 2014.

I have no intention to use cryosaunas frequently any time soon. If they become dirt cheap in the future, I may use them more frequently. For the moment, I will 'stick' to the cheaper and more uncomfortable ('miserability' inducing): cold and ice water immersion and cold showers.

I am excited to experiment with different protocols of cold exposure because I can play with variables such as timing, immediacy/proximity to strength training sessions, frequency, duration (of the dose) and type of exposure, and other factors to intensify the experience. When modulating these variables, my main purpose is to optimize for cold-driven physiologic stress and the adaptive responses that result from it.

Similar to the rest of the stressors discussed in this book, cold and heat stress are very complex and they should always be analyzed in context. The literature on this topic is scant and doubtful from what I can see (should I keep on searching?). This is why I did not get into the interpretation of more studies. In the past I may have been more rushed into using all types of studies (good and bad) to support an argument. However, I think I did not have an adequate capacity for critical interpretation; not to say that I'm much better now. Ok, I may be a little bit better...

In the next chapter I will approach the fields of toxicology and radiation, looking at their relevance to stress and adaptation in human physiology.

I will end this chapter with an anecdotal remark from one of the greatest experimentalists of cold exposure alive, Wim Hof:

"Cold is a merciless, but righteous teacher."

Stress and Adaptation in Physiology

Chapter 6:
Toxicology and Radiation

Much of what I will present in this chapter may come as no surprise to you, in light of what was discussed in earlier chapters.

I will provide details regarding the effects of radiation on living systems and we will look into some studies about this highly disputed topic.

I have to start by saying that over the past 1-2 years many of my beliefs particular to radiation have changed. I used to think that we should try to completely eliminate toxins and other factors perturbing our bodies at all costs. But, in my current view, it does not seem to be like that. Let me review dose response relationships in the context of radiation.

Dose Response Relationships, Radiation, and Radioactivity

Since it was discovered more than a century ago, radioactivity has been the subject of numerous scientific experiments, studies as well as clinical uses. In the early years of the 20th century radiation exposure was being used therapeutically, bearing a lot of promise in treating numerous diseases, including cancers.

Clinicians used mild radium therapy via oral administration of micrograms of radium. This was common practice until a famous millionaire died from radium poisoning; E. M. Byers consumed a large quantity of a radium mixture. This event contributed to the demise of using internal radium for therapeutic purposes [108].

At that time, it was though that no harm from radiation is induced with exposure to doses below a certain threshold. The second half of the 20th century brought into policy the use of the Linear No Threshold model (LNT) that has been adopted across many field. As per Vaiserman (2014):

"The LNT model of radiation carcinogenesis was initially proposed to minimize cancer risk from low-level radiation. This model is based on the following assumptions: every dose, no matter how low, carries with it some cancer risk; risk per unit dose is constant and independent of dose rate (the radiation dose absorbed per unit of time); and risk is additive and increases as dose increases." [108]

As you know from a previous chapter, the LNT model contains flaws; evidence shows how it does not apply in many situations. It has been adopted mostly out of safety concerns (all dose toxins/radiation cause harm), but it may limit the potential benefits from low dose exposure to physiologic perturbations.

Some researchers think that the health impact caused by average levels of radiation (medically induced radiation from diagnosis, background radiation, etc) is lower than that projected by the LNT model:

"Moreover, the LNT hypothesis ignores the fact that life evolved on Earth under conditions of a natural background radiation level, which was significantly higher than today." [108]

As per Karam and Leslie (1999) [109], ~3.5 billion years ago the background radiation levels were three times higher than they are now. Life has evolved under and adapted to extreme conditions. Some researchers think and provide evidence in support of low dose ionizing radiation being beneficial and protective, invoking the biphasic dose-response relationship:

"LD ionizing radiation is among the conditions that bring about biologically beneficial effects by initially causing low level molecular damage, which then leads to the activation of one or more stress response pathways and thereby strengthens homeodynamics." [108]

There have been studies documenting disease risks of radiologists exposed to ionizing radiation ever since the 1940s; these studies reported higher mortality from leukemia, skin cancers and other cancers in radiologists compared to doctors working in other specializations. These associations disappeared as better safety regulations regarding radiation exposure have been implemented after the 1950s. The radio-protection standards of 30,000 mSv/year in 1902 have been changed to 50 mSv/year in 1957 [108].

One sievert (Sv) is a dose equivalent, the result of multiplying the absorbed dose of radiation (Gray - Gy) and a radiation weighing factor. The absorbed dose (in Gy) represents the energy deposited per unit mass and it is used to predict the potential biologic effects of radiation; one Sv is one Gy. One Gy (Gray) is the energy deposition of one Joule per kilogram of tissue [108].

According to Russo and colleagues (2012), cardiologists exposed to long-term low dose radiation exhibit a higher production of hydrogen peroxide (ROS) that may be associated with cellular adaptive responses, such as higher antioxidant capacity and increased apoptosis, which could translate in a greater ability to remove damaged cells [110].

A lot of research data in radiation comes from large epidemiologic and observational studies. One of such studies was conducted between 1980 and 1988. In the Nuclear Shipyard Worker Study, as it was named, researchers looked at workers who have been exposed to external Cobalt-60. They have been divided into three groups:

- high-dose group of 27,872 workers exposed to more than 5 mGy (mSv) during the entire period
- low-dose group of 10,348 workers exposed to less than 5 mGy (mSv) during the entire period
- unexposed group of 32,510 workers.

According to Vaiserman (2014):

"Although this study was designed to search for adverse effects of occupational LD-rate γ radiation, no risks have been reported. Surprisingly, the high-dose exposed workers, on the contrary, demonstrated health benefits compared to the controls. Specifically, the high-dose-exposed cohort had a death rate from all causes 24% lower than the controls. In addition, their death rates from cancer and cardiovascular disease were also significantly lower than those of the controls." [108]

I could not identify inconsistencies in this study or how much other factors would have weighed in, had they been taken into account. This should raise questions and make one appear more skeptical of people/entities fear mongering radiation exposure perils for all dose exposures. Vaiserman (2014) further builds his argument by saying that nuclear workers usually receive less than 100 mSv in a single dose exposure, which is too small to allow for differentiating between cancers induced by radiation and 'naturally' occurring cancers:

"The doses received by nuclear power plant workers fall into this category because exposure is accumulated over many years with an average annual dose about 100 times less than 100 mSv." Since 1983, the U.S. nuclear industry has monitored more than 100,000 radiation workers each year, and no workers have been exposed to more than 50 mSv in a year since 1989 (EPRI 2009)." [108]

One aspect of this matter that seems to make more sense to me is that low dose radiation may elicit positive adaptations to the organism compared to acute or chronic exposure to high levels of radiation. I think that most people today cannot be included in the latter. In support of this theory, Feinendegen and colleagues (2007) explain that:

"The system's response to low-level radiation exposure can evolve from damage to the basic molecular level and also from adaptive responses that may occur on the whole-body level. The balance between damage and protection depends on tissue dose; at single doses below 0.1 Gy, the benefits outweigh the detriments." [111]

Cellular adaptive responses to insults from low-dose radiation include:

- activation of DNA repair pathways
- higher elimination of damaged cells through apoptosis
- activation of stress proteins
- better scavenging of free radicals
- increased immune function
- higher cytokine secretion.

There have been a few studies to support this theory, most of them invoking the concept of hormesis [112, 113, 114]. To understand the importance of dose and duration of exposure, let us look at data involving background radiation.

Vaiserman (2014) [108] discusses about a few large epidemiologic studies that show no risk hazards for populations living in areas of higher background radiation compared to areas of lower background radiation. He reminds about an older, large scale, study from 1976 where researchers reported lower mortality rates from all cancers in states with higher doses of annual radiation [115]. Moreover, according to Vaiserman (2014):

"In a Chinese study, which compared areas with an average radiation exposure of 2.31 mSv/y and areas with 0.96 mSv/y average exposure, the cancer mortality rate was lower in the high background radiation. In another Chinese study, the cancer mortality rate was also lower in the areas with a relatively high background radiation compared to that in areas with lower levels of background radiation. Similarly, in India the cancer incidence and mortality rates were significantly lower in areas with a high background radiation level than in areas with a low level." [115]

Am I trying to argue that radiation exposure is invariably good? Not by far.

I want to point out that every situation should be put into an appropriate context. I am not excluding the possibility that many of the studies that I am citing could contain flaws and may have been written by entities with a certain 'skin' in the game. That is what often happens in the world of research. Nevertheless, this does not mean that all levels of radiation exposure, at any duration and frequency are bad (for human health). We simply do not know for sure.

There may be potential benefits attributed to low-level radiation exposure because this type of perturbation has been shown to induce cellular, tissue, and systemic adaptive responses, in a similar way that other stressors do. I cannot discount all of these studies in light of this argument. Am I skeptical of them? Yes. But I am not disproving them and I am open to explore more studies on radiation and toxic exposure. I think that this can provide important insights for the effects of different dose-response relationships.

To close this short parenthesis, let us look into the proposed molecular mechanisms for adaptive responses to radiation exposure. You may be familiar with them as they are very similar to those elicited by the stressors we've touched upon in this book so far.

Molecular Mechanisms of Radiation Exposure

One mechanism involves **DNA damage response (DDR)**. One of the ways in which DNA can be damaged is through double strand breaks (DSBs), which can lead to genome instability and a potential threat to the viability of the cell [108]. Several papers written by Feinendegen and Pollycove propose that health hazards from radiation exposure are negligible compared to DNA damage from normal metabolic processes [112, 116, 117, 118]. They think that low dose radiation can have a dual effect on DNA.

The first one, the direct effect, is the absorbtion of the energy from radiation to the DNA, leading to structural modifications:

"In addition, the interaction of radiation with water molecules in cells produces water-derived free radicals that lead to DNA damage indirectly. The probability of DNA damage per energy deposition event is relatively low and increases proportionally to the dose absorbed. At background radiation exposure, this damage to DNA is orders of magnitude lower than that from endogenous sources, such as reactive oxygen species (ROSs). In proliferating human cells, the DNA DSBs induced by radiation doses of up to 200 mGy are shown to be completely repaired after 24 hours." [108]

The second effect represents the adaptive protective response against DNA damage which occurs after the exposure to low dose radiation:

"This adaptive protection causes DNA damage prevention and increases DNA repair capacity. It decreases steadily at doses above about 100–200 mGy and is not observed any more after acute exposures of more than about 500 mGy." [108]

I think it is fair to say that this comes in support of my theories that context (dose, duration of exposure, rate/frequency, confounding factors) can make one situation of radiation exposure more beneficial or less detrimental than others.

Another cellular adaptive mechanism of radiation exposure is the **capacity to scavenge free radicals**. Animal models exposed to low-dose radiation show higher activity of the endogenous antioxidant system, which leads to lower ROS-induced oxidation damage. This higher capacity is characterized by increased levels of superoxide dismutase, glutathione, glutathione peroxidase, glutathione reductase, and catalase - enzymes of the endogenous antioxidant system [108]. Another molecular pathway in the adaptive cell response to radiation is Nrf2, which binds to antioxidant response elements (AREs) to activate several defensive mechanisms.

Low dose radiation can induce a slightly increased production of free radicals, which in turn stimulates both the immune system and the antioxidant capacity of the organism. According to Vaiserman (2014):

"In this respect, LD irradiation may be a good alternative to the administration of exogenous antioxidants, which has failed to reduce diseases in clinical trials possibly because there may not have been sufficient bioavailability of antioxidants in the relevant organs to reduce oxidative damage." [108]

Another cellular adaptive mechanism of radiation exposure, also mentioned in an earlier chapter, is the **heat shock response** (HSR), which induces the activation of heat shock proteins (HSPs); some tasks of HSPs involve:

- making sure that other cellular proteins fold correctly
- helping with the refolding of proteins that have been damaged by stressors (in this case, radiation).

Other molecular mechanisms for which there is evidence of beneficial adaptive effects from low dose radiation exposure involve: apoptosis (programmed cell death), autophagy (cellular 'self-eating'), and epigenetic alterations such as DNA methylation, histone acetylation, and different patterns of non-coding RNA expression [108].

While not apparent, it looks more common sense to me that applying a LNT model to radiation and toxic stress from all sources may do more harm than good for public policies. Plus, LNT is not practical because we cannot ensure a complete elimination of environmental or man-induced perturbations (radiation, chemicals like mercury, arsenic, lead, and so on); there will always be some level of residual/marginal exposure.

As I have seen, there are documented positive effects for exposure to low dose insults, making the use of a threshold based rationale more reasonable. A good starting point could be a biphasic dose-response model (low dose stimulation, high dose inhibition).

In light of these thoughts, Vaiserman (2014) remarks:

"Health hazards from ordinarily encountered radiation exposures, such as background radiation, medical x-rays, and so on, are much lower than those given by the LNT-based estimates. Among humans, there is no evidence of a carcinogenic effect for acute irradiation at doses less than 100 mSv and for protracted irradiation at doses less than 500 mSv. Moreover, there is abundant evidence that exposure to LD and LD-rate radiation can be beneficial rather than detrimental and can thereby lead to a hormetic effect." [108]

While there is still too much controversy and concern with respect to the fields of toxicology and radiation, many of such concerns emerge from poor scientific education. Yes, we should be careful with everything that has to do with radiation, but being unrealistically careful may create more harm than good:

"Currently, many authors consider that radiation safety norms are exceedingly restrictive and should be revised to become more realistic and workable. In his recent paper, Jargin (2012) concluded that there are no evidence-based contraindications to fivefold elevation of the total equivalent effective doses to individual members of the public (up to 5 mSv/year) and doubling of the limits for professional exposures." [108, 119]

I am very interested to examine further good research in radiation biology and dose response relationships, not only epidemiologically and retrospectively, but also prospectively (which may raise ethical debates that require special attention). For further study, I recommend reading two recent studies from 2015, one meta-analysis of radon exposure and the risk of developing lung cancer [120] and a review on the molecular mechanisms of low dose ionizing radiation, adaptive responses, bystander effects, radio-resistance, and genomic instability [121].

In the next section, I will briefly discuss mobile phone radiation, and in the last section of this chapter I will provide examples of human physiologic adaptations (increased tolerance) to arsenic exposure.

Mobile Phone Radiation

Research on the biologic effects of mobile phone radiation is a fairly new field because mobile phones have invaded our existence just recently - one to two decades ago. I think there is too much speculation for the potential negative health effects of phone radiation without enough consistent and strong evidence to support such arguments. This view is different from the one I adopted in a previous book, *The Testosterone Protocol*. Have I changed my perspective?

In part, yes. I think that the modest evidence I reviewed back then was not put under enough scrutiny. Additionally, I think I may have been influenced by 'strong' personalities (let me avoid the use of the word 'gurus') in my past views, without efficiently investigating some of their claims. I used to think that we should protect ourselves from any type and any dose of radiation coming from our phones. I also thought that nobody should ever keep their phones in their front pockets because this will have a massive negative impact on their reproductive health.

I still think that some of these concerns are reasonable in appropriate circumstances: mobile phone radiation exists; whether or not it has biological effects still remains to be elucidated. Poorly conducted and highly interpretable studies claim that mobile phone radiation causes negative biologic effects; Personally, I still did not encounter decent research on this topic to show clear biologic effects in humans, which is why I try to keep an open mind and look forward to upcoming research; this is different from the inflexible and one sided perspective I used to hold.

Here, I will discuss the following: a review article from 2015 on the physiological and pathophysiological considerations of mobile phone radiation and an article written by Steven Novella, clinical neurologist and editor of the *Science Based Medicine* website. I consider Professor Novella a strong example of critical thinking and a person that I follow closely.

Radiation from mobile devices comes in the form of electromagnetic emissions and can interfere with brain signals because they are similar in oscillation [122]. High power density levels may induce local thermal effects (heating of the area in close proximity to the source of electromagnetic radiation (EMR)). However, there are also, less understood, effects that occur at lower power density levels without the induction of local heating.

Worldwide safety standards have been created based on these thermal effects.

"For the mobile phones, ICNIRP 1998 guidelines restrict spatial peak of microwave exposure to 2 W/Kg SAR values averaged over 10 g of tissue for 6 minutes." [122]

In numerous studies and scientific reports, researchers discuss adverse effects of EMR such as male infertility, brain tumors, as well as reduced immune function [122]. According to Nageswari (2015):

"There are equal number of conflicting reports in literature regarding EMR exposure and brain tumors. A comprehensive review concludes 'overall the studies published to date do not demonstrate an increased risk within approximately 10 years of use for any tumor of the brain or any other head tumor'." [122]

Moreover:

"Another review summarizes that there is "enough data to convince that long-term exposure to low intensity EMR below the ICNIRP guidelines can promote cancer development". However the time limit for exposure has been suggested as more than 10 years." [122]

10 years? We've only been using mobile phones extensively since the introduction of the smartphone (circa 2006), which is barely 10 years ago. This alone is a heavy factor that could potentially invalidate past research in light of emerging research. There are other numerous factors that have failed to be accounted for in past studies, and which need to be considered appropriately in the future. According to Nageswari (2015):

"For conducting epidemiological studies, some of the difficulties experienced are obtaining unexposed controls or cohorts, follow up of the cohorts, actual dose measurement for exposure assessment in case-

control studies, inaccuracy, recall bias and selective non response in recall of phone use by mobile phone users, long induction times, long latencies (the effects we observe now are of analogue phones that are no longer used) and the rarity of observed malignancies, variable ways of using the phone by the user i.e. left or right ear, head sets/speaker/blue tooth etc." [122]

When you acknowledge the state of the matter with these factors in mind, you may understand the existence of potential flaws and inaccuracies in previous studies. Personally, I currently try to do that. While I do not completely disregard what has been published so far, I am moving away from the single-sided perspective that I used to have: that my phone and Wi-Fi router are going to kill me.

Novella (2016) is in the camp of people who think that a causal relationship between cell phones and cancers is really low. First, Novella differentiates between mobile phone radiation (non-ionizing) and ionizing radiation - which has the capacity to perturb DNA and induce mutations [123]. Please remember what I wrote previously in the book: not all doses of ionizing radiation induce negative effects.

Unlike ionizing radiation, non-ionizing radiation does not have the power to break chemical bonds, as per Novella (2016):

"Physicists in particular like this physics argument and conclude that non-ionizing radiation is of no possible health risk. Physicians, however, coming from a biological point of view sometimes argue that biology is complex and we cannot always anticipate all the possible indirect mechanisms of harm. Non-ionizing radiation, for example, may heat tissue causing some indirect harmful effect. Even this mechanism, however, is questionable as the local heating caused by cell phone use is probably insignificant compared to other daily factors." [123]

Novella (2016) also mentions the existence of questionable (he calls them dubious) studies that point to the possible correlations between cell phones and any type of cancer, but in his view and according to the bulk of research, there is no such correlation. In fact, he points toward a decreasing trend in brain cancer incidence in the last 30 years (0.2% per year), referencing to government data (statistics), publicly available through SEER (Surveillance, Epidemiology, and End Results Program) [124].

While concerns regarding radiation and toxic exposure are legit, I think that we are currently over-concerned and we do not have enough good data to support our concerns. It is safe to say, like always, that much more research is further needed to gain better insight into the issue.

Leaving mobile phone radiation aside, let me turn to another facet of stress adaptation in humans - a good example showing evolution at work.

Human Adaptation to Arsenic Exposure

The land and the drinking water in the northern part of the Argentinean Andes have a higher concentration of arsenic compared to other regions such as Peru, which is in its immediate proximity. The groundwater near San Antonio de los Cobres, the Argentinean village in the Andes, contains about 200 micrograms of arsenic per liter, which is approximately 20 times higher than what is considered acceptable by the World Health Organization.

In a paper from 2015, Schlebusch and colleagues found that inhabitants of the Andean region posses a unique arsenic metabolism characterized by efficient methylation and excretion of dimethylated arsenic and a reduced excretion of the highly toxic monomethylated arsenic. Here's what they did:

"We genotyped women from this population for 4,301,332 single nucleotide polymorphisms (SNPs) and found a strong association between the AS3MT (arsenic [+3 oxidation state] methyltransferase) gene and mono- and dimethylated arsenic in urine, suggesting that AS3MT functions as the major gene for arsenic metabolism in humans." [125]

Their study reveals strong genetic differentiation near AS3MT in Andeans compared to the Peruvians exposed to much lower levels of arsenic. This is probably the first clearly documented case of such selection in humans. We know of other examples of selection in different populations, such as: lactase persistence in some African and European populations, CNV (copy number variation) in AMY1 (amylase gene) allowing some populations to better digest starchy foods, selection for genes that provide resistance to cholera and malaria, selection for genes that enable better adaptation to living at higher altitudes, etc.

In their conclusion, Schlebusch et al. (2015) note that:

"Our data show that adaptation to tolerate the environmental stressor arsenic has likely driven an increase in the frequencies of protective variants of AS3MT, providing the first evidence of human adaptation to a toxic chemical." [125]

Similar reports have been created based on this study [126, 127]. Independently, other researchers conducted a genome wide association study, this time in Bangladeshi people, of arsenic related metabolism and toxicity phenotypes. In their analyses they also looked at variants in the same or similar genes that can influence (and increase) the risk of developing arsenic toxicity when exposed to arsenic (these would be the 'negative' variants). According to Pierce and colleagues (2012):

"Using array-based genome-wide gene expression data, we show that several of our lead genetic variants are associated with expression of

AS3MT and neighboring gene C10orf32, providing a potential mechanism by which 10q24.32 variants influence arsenic metabolism and toxicity. Knowledge of variation in this region and associated biological processes could be used to develop intervention and pharmacological strategies aimed at preventing large numbers of arsenic-related deaths in arsenic-exposed populations." [128]

It may seem common sense to think that such adaptations (selection) to this environmental stressor have developed through time, similar to other adaptations that I mentioned a few paragraphs ago. These adaptations represent powerful examples of how people living in different environments can respond differently to perturbing agents. Hence, for every strategy, context primes.

I personally think that any protocol you may follow (whether it's your diet, sleep, exercising, radiation and toxic chemical exposure, supplementation, thermal stress, and other stressors), you may be better off if you individualize your strategy by including as many factors and variables from your life and environment as possible. General recommendations can serve as a good starting point; but that is the only thing they should represent. It is my hope that the maturation of the genomics field and the emergence of more genome wide association studies (GWAS) will provide a clearer message to support this rationale.

The following chapter is an accelerated overview of aging and healthy lifespan, as seen through the lenses of physiologic stress and adaptation.

Chapter 7:
Aging and Longevity

It is not easy to approach the topics of aging and longevity from a solid scientific perspective. How is it then that so many studies are published in peer reviewed journals every year and so many entities, either individuals or companies, promise the next compound or strategy to 'eliminate' aging in humans?

First of all, it is not only I but also others (who are much smarter than me) who considered that most of the published research is flawed, to put it so very mildly [129]. Profiting from the lack of scientific literacy of the wide public and exploiting human innate cognitive biases, researchers can publish what appears to be a good study to support any claim they want. Framing and statistical manipulations are two of the numerous deceptive practices. Thus, the little current good research that may exist with respect to aging may hide behind this insurmountable noise of non-sense.

In my view, the majority of good evidence that we have about improving longevity in humans is theoretical. Anecdotal evidence, meta-analyses and epidemiologic studies are helpful, but they do not provide strong associations in support of improving our longevity. I do not want to appear pessimistic, but the topic of longevity seems unbearably complex, especially in humans.

While there may be pathways that are directly associated with aging and act in a 'clear' direction in model organisms (simpler than humans), that cannot be said about us. For example, manipulating the IIS axis (Insulin and IGF-1) in simple organisms can extend lifespan several times [130].

Conducting experiments in organisms that live longer is troublesome. One of the major barriers is represented by the unfeasibility of such approach. With simpler organisms that normally live from days to months, researchers can design strategies, generate hypotheses, conduct studies and make observations in relatively short periods of time. To design and conduct aging experiments in humans would require decades, if not longer. Plus, multiple independent studies would have to try to replicate these experiments.

I am not saying that it is impossible, but I think it is highly improbable that solid answers with respect to longevity in humans will come from such studies. Moreover, I am not dismissing the research done in simpler organisms. On the contrary, I think such experiments are extremely valuable because they provide suggestions and insights that we could apply and observe in more complex organisms. And this is what I intend to do in this short chapter: look at scatter data from various organisms and cell cultures and hypothesize for potential human applications (direct or for research purposes).

One thought that I become more confident about, as time passes, is with regards to the fields of molecular genetics, genomics, and nanotechnology. I think it is possible that our answers for positively manipulating lifespan may come from technology or a combination of biology and technology; biological manipulations alone may be too complicated or too difficult to implement for this purpose; of course, I am merely speaking from the top of my mind here.

Let me approach the aging topic from a perspective that you are already familiar with, that of homeostasis and homeodynamics, and see how adaptive stressors could fit into this picture.

According to the **mechanistic principle of longevity**, aging represents accumulated molecular damage (in DNA, proteins, cells, and so on) that cannot be repaired or managed efficiently [131].

By some theories, it is thought that the essential lifespan of humans is limited to a few extra years past the maturation of our reproductive function. Survival beyond this essential life-span may thus be accompanied by progressive and cumulative molecular damage.

Recall that homeodynamics extends homeostasis (our internal equilibrium of chemical and biological processes) by stating that equilibrium is never maintained for long, despite the ever present tendency to return to it. Factors of physiologic stress perturb homeostasis; our body's response is to return to equilibrium. In light of this, Rattan (2008) affirms that:

"The process of aging is primarily characterized by a progressive shrinking of homeodynamic space in terms of increased molecular heterogeneity, which leads to increased vulnerability, onset of diseases, and eventual death." [131]

Thus, through homeodynamics our bodies try to ensure healthy aging:

"The progressive failure of homeodynamics leads to the physiological malfunctioning manifested as a general functional decline, diseases and ultimate death." [132]

Hence, strategies that may slow the development of age related diseases and which may improve longevity should focus on enlarging the homeodynamic space, the window (if I may) in which we can efficiently distance from homeostasis, through factors of physiologic stress. Increasing the homeodynamic space should enable the ability to live in a varied range of environments and to withstand perturbations from more stressors. It should also improve our capacity to efficiently repair the damage incurred by such physiologic perturbing factors. Always seeking physiologic comfort can, thus, be debilitating and incapacitating because our biologic system is never challenged beyond a narrow homeostatic window.

You may not be surprised that stressors could favor such homeodynamic adaptations. Mild to moderate, but not chronic, exposure to acute stressors, may support healthy aging. We have already discussed them at length throughout the book, which is why I'm only going to briefly mention them here.

Certain natural and synthetic dietary compounds may have biological effects, as they act on one or more pathways involved in stress and adaptive responses. Vitamins, minerals, phytochemicals, and other trace elements that are present in food, but not in supplemental form, have been show to elicit such effects; examples include: resveratrol, alpha lipoic acid, curcumin, etc.

Dietary restriction in the forms of chronic calorie restriction without malnutrition, intermittent calorie restriction, intermittent fasting and prolonged fasting may also represent beneficial stressors for healthy lifespan. According to Kyriazis (2010):

"Long periods of dietary restriction have been found to increase the health and maximum life span of many organisms. However, it appears that it is not only the duration of DR that is relevant but also the frequency and timing of the dieting episodes. This is called intermittent fasting (IF). IF upregulates BDNF and improves signaling of enzymes involved with glucose regulation or with cardiovascular function." [135]

Intermittent fasting has been shown to upregulate proteolysis, suppress glycolysis and lead to the generation of

165

fewer methylglyoxal molecules - which is responsible for abnormal bonding of enzymes and proteins. Accordingly, lymphocytes taken from the blood of people with low BMI showed a higher capacity to repair DNA [135].

It follows that non-linearity (moving away from regularity and consistency) can be a beneficial implementation of dietary stress that may favor healthy aging. To be more specific, as per Kyriazis (2010):

"It may be suggested that periods of fasting should be followed by periods of overeating. This model closely follows phylogenetic mechanisms designed to help our ancestors cope with successive periods of famine and overabundance of food. It may also be claimed that having meals at irregular times during the day may resemble a more natural pattern of feeding and could act as a type of nutritional stimulus to the digestive apparatus, with positive results. In this case, the irregularity and nonmonotony of the meals would act as a mildly stressful hormetic event." [135]

I do not think I could have described it better than that. Another component from the category of dietary stress involves alcohol consumption. The research that I looked at so far is inclined in the direction that one may be better off not consuming alcohol at all. Some research supports benefiting from low to moderate alcohol consumption, but the effects have been observed in non-healthy people.

"The moderate use of alcohol as a hormetic poison has a beneficial effect in unhealthy older men only and no effect on healthy cohorts." [135]

My current view of this issue may be limited since I did not read extensively on the topic, which is why I do not have a strong opinion about this.

While I may be more reserved, others may be more liberate and supportive for moderate alcohol consumption. As per Rattan (2008:

"Dietary intake of moderate amounts of ethanol has been shown to have memory enhancing beneficial effects in mice. In the case of humans, consumption of moderate amounts of alcohol, combined with other positive lifestyle factors, has been associated with fourfold reduction in mortality." [131]

This shouldn't be considered as licensing for alcohol consumption. In my own perspective, I would favor infrequent and random ingestion of small to moderate doses of alcohol. To be more specific: 1-2 medium size glasses of wine or 2-3 oz. of hard alcohol once every couple of days (5-6 days), or even more random: today, 5 days later, then 3 days later, then 8 days, etc; hopefully, you get the point (of randomness).

As of current, I am not in favor of frequent (daily, every 2-3 days) alcohol consumption, even in moderate doses. If consumed at night, it perturbs sleep; if consumed accompanying meals, it interferes with digestion. If you do it infrequently, your body may be more able to respond adaptively to such perturbation, but if you do it frequently it may be detrimental over the long term (even in moderate doses). Keep in mind, these are my current anecdotal thoughts.

Exercise done acutely and intensely, but not chronically, may serve as an adaptive stressor. Exercise generates reactive oxygen species, which then stimulate *"antioxidant repair mechanisms together with DNA repair and protein degradation enzyme activation, all of which are affected during aging."* [135]

The dose and the frequency are important. As pointed out by Radak and colleagues (2008) in a widely cited paper:

"Therefore, chronic stressors could be very dangerous since the resting period, which is obligatory for recovery and efficient stress response, is missing. Using extremely long-duration exercise as an example, such as 18–24 consecutive hours of running or swimming, even in superbly trained individuals, the body can suffer serious "exhaustion" which could jeopardize the health of the individuals." [134]

They go by explaining that in overtraining, adaptation fails to occur, primarily because of an incomplete recovery from the dose of exercise received. I would assume that they refer to overtraining in all types and flavors of exercise, endurance or resistance. Fatigue also seems to be important in the process of adaptation:

"The level of fatigue is important, since extreme fatigue could cause very significant cellular alterations, even irreversible ones, and the recovery period after extreme fatigue could be too long, which makes it difficult to establish an exercise regimen." [134]

Both extremes of the exercise spectrum, overtraining and inactivity appear to impair and decrease physiologic function, thus putting a biological system's response to exercise under a U-shaped curve. Moreover, as per Kyiriazis (2010):

"One way of enhancing both physical and mental inputs and increasing complex neuronal and muscular interactions is to use different types of unusual, nonmonotonic, mild exercises performed at irregular and ever-changing times. This irregularity exposes the nervous, musculoskeletal, and cardiovascular systems to new and challenging stimuli that upregulate their function." [135]

Leslie (2005) makes some good points in a *Science* article on how we could use stress to fortify our physiologic condition. She starts by presenting the literature on model organisms subjected to stress and their ability to respond adaptively:

Stress and Adaptation in Physiology

"A stack of studies has documented salutary effects from moderate doses of heavy metals, radiation, high temperatures, stronger-than-normal gravity, and other torturous stimuli." [133]

When it comes to applications in humans, things might get more complicated, at least from a research standpoint:

"Human studies rely on individuals exposed accidentally or for another purpose, such as shipyard workers irradiated on the job, who suffered fewer cancers than did unexposed workers." [133]

In a somewhat contradictory argument, Kyriazis (2010) notes:

"Whereas mild radiation stress produces benefits in experimental conditions, a wider study of 400,000 nuclear plant workers showed that exposure to mild radiation actually decreases life span." [135]

We have to be careful in interpreting and extrapolating data, especially if we cannot benefit from the availability of human studies specifically designed for such purposes.

As I have discussed earlier, it is ethically and methodologically challenging to conduct long-term human trials that involve the administration of physiologic perturbations. We can look retrospectively at epidemiologic data and also at disaster survival data (chemical and radiation accidents, for example). But is this enough?

In designing such trials, there are numerous challenges that we may need to face, including:

- subjects responding differently to the same dose of stressor
- finding the effective dose
- finding the effective frequency and duration of exposure

- assessing and understanding tolerance buildup and the requirement for a constant re-assessment of dose, frequency and duration of exposure.

Leslie (2005) points out that:

"Even if we can overcome these challenges, another obstacle looms: convincing residents of the modern world, who are increasingly loath to put down their burgers and cake, that therapeutic suffering has value." [133]

We do not have to solve all these research related challenges to immediately create practical and helpful strategies in our daily lives.

We have countless of anecdotal examples where deliberately subjecting oneself to physiologic stressors can aid human condition in the long run. It then remains a matter of individual choice and preferences to do it or not. I am inclined to think that a healthy majority of people are not in favor of deliberate exposure to stressors - as it necessarily implies physiologic and psychologic discomfort.

To reiterate one of my previous arguments:

I am (currently) confident that appropriate exposure to stressors could help us age better and live longer, but I think that the solution(s) to the aging riddle is/are likely to come from a combination of biology and technology (biotech) because biological manipulations alone may be too weak or insufficient for this purpose.

Stress and Adaptation in Physiology

Chapter 8:
Cognitive Stress and the Concept of Anti-Fragility

By pretending you can remove all risks, you lose the ability to grow from facing those risks.

Steven Bratman

Most of the literature on stress (that I am familiar with) deals with psychologic stress and resilience. There are countless books, both popular (for the public at large, mostly self-help non-scientific books) and scientific books (including textbooks) on this topic, while so very few explore the physiologic particularities of stress and adaptive responses. Yet, part of our biochemistry (as I see it now) is substantially characterized and driven by these mechanisms.

Thus, one of my main reasons to write this book came from my inability to find as much scientific literature as I wanted on the topic of physiologic stress. To complete my homework for this book, I had to study the works of scientific pioneers from a multitude of fields. I have been presenting them to you throughout the book. My comments, interventions and personal anecdotes may have aided the understanding of the book, or so I hope; though, I have to recognize that I did not protect you from exposure to scientific terminology.

I want to dedicate part of this last chapter to an interesting perspective on psychologic stress. I will then finish with my current practical formulation to benefit from physiologic and psychologic stress, and with a philosophical view inspired by Nicholas Nassim Taleb's concept of anti-fragility.

Adaptive and Maladaptive Psychologic Stress

James Baldwin, American writer, was able to view deep into the essence of the nature of life. Here's what he writes in 1961:

Stress and Adaptation in Physiology

"Any real change implies the breakup of the world as one has always known it, the loss of all that gave one an identity, the end of safety. And at such a moment, unable to see and not daring to imagine what the future will now bring forth, one clings to what one knew, or thought one knew; to what one possessed or dreamed that one possessed." [138]

Baldwin further elaborates:

"Yet, it is only when one is able, without bitterness or self-pity, to surrender a dream one has long cherished or a privilege one has long possessed that one is set free—one has set oneself free—for higher dreams, for greater privileges." [138]

We all know this, right? Sure we do. However, you should not be surprised how so very few people can objectively detach from their own persona and adopt a proactive approach through such a burdensome process that change is - either physiologic, psychologic or both. Change, in and of itself, implies discomfort; humans are comfortable creatures with a tendency for inertia - that of not deviating far from a central point (homeostasis).

Here I want to introduce, interpret, and build atop of the perspective of stress and adaptation of Dr. Martha Stark, who teaches clinical psychiatry at Harvard Medical School and who is a teacher and supervising analyst at Massachusetts Institute for Psychoanalysis [137].

In one of her recent writings, Stark (2014) discusses about optimal frustration: *"that will provide the therapeutic leverage needed to provoke, after initial disruption, eventual revitalization of the system at a higher level of functionality and adaptive capacity."* [137]

The disruption she mentions can be psychological, physiological, or both, and can be provoked by stressors including, but not limited to:

"- the accumulation of metabolic waste products in the body;
- an interpersonal disappointment;
- exposure to the aluminum found in antiperspirants or the mercury
found in dental amalgams;
- psychological, physical, or sexual abuse;
- contact with a carcinogenic pesticide (such as the insect repellent
DEET);
- the loss of a parent;
- or the ingestion of endocrine disruptors (such as the phthalates found
in plastic bottles)." [137]

Maladaptive stress or the inability to adapt from stress involves, in her view, too much of a bad thing and not enough good of another thing. Relevant examples are:

- too much oxidative stress, not enough antioxidant capacity
- too much criticism, not enough acceptance
- too many antibiotics, not enough probiotics
- too many anxiety provoking thoughts, not enough anxiety reducing interventions
- etc [137].

I think this view goes one step beyond the argument that any stimuli can be harmful if overdosed and/or delivered chronically. Thus, finding the 'optimal frustration', or an optimal dose of stress for psychological growth, remains a constant challenge for the individual.

But what exactly can be included in the category of psychologic stressor? Does it always imply a pathologic state? Are we always talking about cognitive stress particular to a disease/disordered state? Or is it that healthy people can self-administer cognitive stressors at certain doses, frequencies, and durations of exposure to make their minds more resilient? I will get to this in a moment...

As pointed by Stark (2014), we do not know the exact details of 'the' optimal dose of psychologic stress; it could differ from one individual to another. What we can do and what she advises psychotherapists do is something along the following lines:

"We just do the best we can to buy low and sell high and then make whatever adjustments we need to optimize the return on our portfolio." [137]

Simply put: do the best you can with what you have; and then adjust. The state of health of a biological system is a matter of continuously responding and adjusting to environmental perturbation; a matter of self-organization to ever-changing homeostatic set points [137].

Building on top of the concepts of poison-medication, a stressful mental input could be good, bad, or neutral, depending on the particularities of its dosage. There are many reasonable exceptions to this: it could be difficult to include the loss of a close one in the category of positive mental input regardless of the 'dose' (how much it hurts); however, one can always take something good out of any experience; the form of 'good' in this instance remains contextual and subjective.

The Development of Mental Potential

Cognitive stress is not particular to dysfunctional or disordered states. Healthy people can make use of mental stressors to build psychologic resilience. Delivering a good dose of mental stress at a certain frequency can increase mental sharpness, reduce cognitive decline, as well as counteract brain aging [137]. Similar to athletes improving their physical fitness by self-administering doses of interval training, you and I can self-administer mental challenges to enhance our mental 'fitness'. In such context, the brain is perceived like a muscle, which without frequent and deliberate exercise will atrophy.

But what are some examples of such mental challenges? Martha Stark (2014) comes up with a few ideas:

"...any mental exercise requiring deliberate and concentrated effort (e.g., active repetition, focused attention, learning a new skill or a new language, reflection, or meditation) will promote mental agility and delay age-related decline in mental capacity." [137]

I could further elaborate on this by saying that exposing yourself to anything new (environmental richness) that takes your mind out of auto-pilot can extend the homeostatic space of the mind:

- walk/drive home via a different route than usual
- wake up at odd hours
- read a book or listen to a podcast on a topic that you are not familiar with
- try to meet people from backgrounds or with preoccupations far different from yours
- visit new places
- hope you get the point; examples are unlimited.

As per Stark (2014), our brains get stimulated when we expose ourselves to new, different, unusual or unexpected situations and stimuli. Our brain loves variety and novelty, or that which is different to habitual life:

Whereas routine activity (i.e., doing the same thing day in and day out) can deaden the brain, spicing things up by introducing variety into one's daily routines can provide the optimally stressful challenge needed to activate underused neural pathways and connections, thereby making the brain more fit and flexible. [137]

An interesting and unconventional mental stressor could be delivered through the deliberate creation of cognitive dissonance. Exposing your mind to thoughts that are different from your established 'beliefs' creates mental conflict - an unpleasant mental state. Stark (2014) provides a few good examples of dissonance:

" *You know that your need to keep what really matters to you hidden, incommunicado, private means that you will never really be able to have deep connection or real intimacy with anyone; but you have been betrayed so many times in the past that you are not now sure that you will ever again dare to open your heart. You're coming to understand that your anger can put people off, but you tell yourself that you have a right to be as angry as you want because of how much you have had to suffer over the years.* "[137]

Dissonance is not a sustainable state of mind because your brain's tendency is for minimal energy consumption; cognitive dissonance 'burns' a lot of energy. As you reach mental resolution, your current conclusions may have renewed your established beliefs; I assume and hope that most of the time when you create cognitive dissonance, your renewed beliefs are better than your former.

Dissonance and the types of environmental enrichment that I mentioned above require active attention and input from your brain; evolutionarily speaking, your mind has to absorb novelty and new stimuli and interpret them appropriately, otherwise your survival might be at stake; I am exaggerating for the sake of understanding.

It has been said, anecdotally and in research, that the brain and the mind operate on the principle of least resistance: preserving energy is a priority. Novelty and new stimuli require higher consumption of energy and an overall increased activity of the mental system. Most obvious, such mental stimuli create discomfort in an effort to return one-self to that which they are most familiar with. In comfort, the brain uses the least amount of energy; our habitual lives are testimony for this argument.

Personal side note: cognitive inertia, or the lack of deliberate mental challenge, may lead to an inability to grow your mind.

Taking our brains out of comfort, exposing ourselves to new stimuli and to mental stressors, seems like an appropriate strategy to use in our efforts to grow mentally. Logically speaking, how could one grow from comfort? How could one's brain and mind become more resilient if they are only exposed to habitual life, where the brain is minimally challenged?

I know, through personal experience, that all these strategies of stressing the mind, all these tactics of taking yourself out of comfort, are extremely uncomfortable; they create physiologic and psychologic unease - an increased state of unpleasantness. Even knowing this, I often find it hard to deliberately induce physical and mental discomfort; what pushes me beyond inertia is my confidence that this (discomfort) is one of the very few ways in which I can grow physically and mentally. I also know that most people are not willing to go through it.

Going off topic for a brief moment, I think that the entire non-sensical literature of self-development can be boiled down to one phrase: remove yourself from comfort.

Getting back on topic, most of the mental stimuli I mentioned above may increase the levels of BDNF - brain derived neurotrophic factor, which is like a fertilizer for brain cells, prompting them to grow quicker and stronger:

"BDNF supports the survival of existing neurons, fosters the generation of new neurons from neural stem cells (i.e., neurogenesis), and

encourages the development of new and more flexible connections between neurons (i.e., synaptic plasticity)." [137]

I have to re-emphasize one of the most important aspects of stress and adaptation: it is the dose, duration, and frequency of exposure to the stressor that can turn it from medication to poison. Always searching and adjusting for the right dose, then, becomes a priority. Too little of a stressor may provide low or no opportunity for adaptation and growth, while too much of a stressor may be maladaptive and detrimental. This requires constant and active vigilance.

Antifragility and Some of My Current Tactics

Statistician, essayist, risk analyst, scholar and former trader, Nicholas Nassim Taleb is one character that marked my current life perspective with his works: *The Black Swan: The Impact of the Highly Improbable* and *Anti-Fragile: Things That Gain From Disorder* [143, 144].

Anti-fragility, as described by Taleb (2012), takes stress and adaptation to a new level. Becoming physiologically and psychologically antifragile, if I may, does not only make you more resilient, but it allows you to grow from stress; it allows you to thrive on stress [144]. According to Carver (1998):

"Thriving (physical or psychological) may reflect decreased reactivity to subsequent stressors, faster recovery from subsequent stressors, or a consistently higher level of functioning. Psychological thriving may reflect gains in skill, knowledge, confidence, or a sense of security in personal relationships." [139]

We do not like to be uncertain about something because this creates mental unease and a sense of insecurity. In our lives, most of us steer clear from uncertainty; we succumb to comfort; the world we live in is, however, highly uncertain. With such self-imposed incapacitation, we reduce our ability to 'survive' unpredictable events. Thriving is, then, out of discussion.

As per Greco and Roger (2003), uncertainty is a powerful mental stressor [140]. Are there ways in which we could exploit uncertainty to gain from unexpected and unpredictable negative situations?

To put it more philosophically, in the words of Taleb:

"Wind extinguishes a candle and energizes fire. Likewise with randomness, uncertainty, chaos: you want to use them, not hide from them. You want to be the fire and wish for the wind. We just don't want to just survive uncertainty, to just about make it. We want to survive uncertainty and, in addition— like a certain class of aggressive Roman Stoics— have the last word." [142]

As we have learned throughout the book, trying to eliminate stress and stressors can be counterproductive and can make us more fragile in the face of physical and mental challenges; I fail to understand the logic of us doing it so consistently and with such propensity.

In Taleb's reasoning, the opposite of fragile is not robust, resilient or unbreakable; it is antifragile: that which actually gains from disorder, chaos, disaster, and any other conceivable perturbing situation. While the resilient resists perturbation and remains the same, the antifragile thrives on perturbation.

Simple examples that illustrate antifragility:

"In the case of evolution, nature uses disorder to grow stronger. Occasional starvation or going to the gym also makes you stronger, because you subject your body to stressors and gain from them." [141]

I hope you understand that I am talking about something that most of us intuitively fear of and try to stay away from.

How could one love error, randomness, and uncertainty, when we are, naturally, so eager to be correct, consistent, regular and habitual? We strive for order in our lives. Yet:

"The antifragile loves randomness and uncertainty, which also means— crucially— a love of errors, a certain class of errors." [142]

Applying or trying to perceive nutrition and modern diseases through the lenses of antifragility, Taleb (2012) notes:

"Diabetes and many similar modern ailments seem to be associated with a lack of randomness in feeding and the absence of the stressor of occasional starvation." [142]

In other words, our lives are too predictable, too ordered and structured, and too habitual. A lack of randomness and volatility may predispose us to detrimental physiologic and psychologic outcomes. A biologic system deprived of anti-fragility is likely going to suffer:

"Crucially, if antifragility is the property of all those natural (and complex) systems that have survived, depriving these systems of volatility, randomness, and stressors will harm them. They will weaken, die, or blow up." [142]

Moreover, according to Taleb (2012):

"We have been fragilizing the economy, our health, political life, education, almost everything...by suppressing randomness and volatility. Just as spending a month in bed (preferably with an unabridged version of War and Peace and access to The Sopranos' entire eighty-six episodes) leads to muscle atrophy, complex systems are weakened, even killed, when deprived of stressors." [142]

One of the tragedies of the modern world, Taleb (2012) thinks, is the lack of people with skin in the game, or, in other words, the abundance of non-risk takers [142]. Without getting into self-development non-sense, I shortly argument that most of us favor risk avoidance, whether it is about nutrition, exercise, relationships, career, family, you name it. Our natural inclination towards comfort may prevent us from rising above mediocrity.

Gaining from Disorder

These concepts may look good on paper and while the majority of our modern society does not deliberately self-subject to stressors and, by extrapolation, to anything that has to do with anti-fragility, there are some exceptions.

Even though I've recently grown aware of the intricacies of the scientific method and the human innate susceptibility to logical fallacies and cognitive biases (our inborn flaws), I still share a deep respect for those who walk their talk, the people who do what they preach without necessarily being backed by rigorous scientific evidence.

After all, it is so easy to appear very knowledgeable on a subject matter today, given the free availability of information. Yet, individuals who not only talk, but also apply what they preach, are distinguishable. When Nassim Taleb was asked about how he applies the principles of anti-fragility in his life, his response was:

"I lift stones and do weightlifting. I don't go to the doctor except when I'm very ill, and when I go to India, I drink a drop of local water. Things like this harness the body's antifragility. I have never had personal debt and never will. I also picked a profession in which I am antifragile, because any attack makes me stronger. When I write about something, I have skin in the game, and I have benefited more from attacks on The Black Swan than been harmed by them..." [141]

His entire philosophy cannot be grasped in a few paragraphs, which is why I recommend, if one is interested, to read his books on randomness and antifragility.

What is it that I do in my life particular to stress and adaptation?

As I have previously noted, only recently I became more knowledgeable about the scientific method, about statistical manipulations in research studies, and about our inborn mental flaws. The concepts of cognitive biases and logical fallacies are also very complex. By default, we are not creatures of reason, but creatures of rationalization. Our mind is set to find patterns in meaningless data; we are gullible, we do not seek arguments that follow reason; instead, we use rationalization through retrofitting and hindsight to enforce our already established beliefs.

Changing one's mind is effortful and discomforting. We do not like such mental challenges. Sticking to one's beliefs implies little discomfort, which is why seeking evidence to fit into our established beliefs and discarding the opposite, is what we mostly do. These and countless others features of our mental flaws are what prevent us from becoming creatures of reason, critical thinkers if I may.

The brain we are born with is faulty for modern day use. We are not good thinkers by nature, we are driven by habits. A good critical mind is developed through deliberate practice, same as you build muscle with resistance training. Becoming aware of our mental flaws is the first step...

Practicing critical thinking everyday through meta-cognition - thinking about your thinking and your thought processes -, through questioning one's thoughts, through objective analyses of the arguments one is presented with, and through numerous other strategies is an effortful strategy to upgrade one's mind from its primate nature.

Building on top of these arguments, I will say that I currently hold no definitive personal life strategy. Moving from a former more rigid self, I seek to change my life approach whenever I am presented with good arguments to do so.

Nonetheless, there are some defining lines that I currently follow and that seem to have persisted through time, while other of my life strategies have changed or have been completely removed from my life. Thus, whatever follows in the next paragraphs should be taken as 'current' strategy, subjective to change. Should you take anything good from it? That is up to you.

First, let's talk about nutritional stress. I do not believe in a general diet to be prescribed to the majority of people. I used to believe that the ketogenic diet falls into this category. But I don't think that's the case anymore. There are many ways to do the ketogenic diet wrong and there are so many people who do it wrong, failing to take something good out of it. This applies to the other extreme of the diet spectrum as well: so many people fail when following low fat diets.

Few, from what I've seen, are successful in their approach in any dietary context. I think that diets fail because of the limitations and the rigidity they impose (not allowing you to eat the forbidden food may increase your desire to eat it).

I would say that such limitations (don't eat carbs, stay away from fat) can be good temporarily, but folks seem unable to limit themselves. Thence, it is not necessarily the rigid nature of a diet that's wrong; it's the fact that one cannot discipline him/herself enough to stay within the boundaries of these limitations.

Extreme diets, in my view, can be most beneficial to people who are metabolically deranged. Taking away a perturbation/stressor with the purpose of resensitizing a biological system to it can be a reasonable strategy. Completely removing sugar, temporarily, from the diet of an insulin resistant person is reasonable to allow that person to restore insulin sensitivity. Whether the 'temporary' nature of such a strategy should become 'constant' is a very contextual and individual matter. I would say that chronic deprivation of a stimulus is a strategy meant to fail.

Thus, extreme diets can be most efficient to those that are far from physiologic normalcy. As soon as a limiting diet approaches its goals, an individual could start moving away from rigidity and start becoming more flexible, by delivering unpredictable dietary stimuli to the body. Let me exemplify.

For example, someone who managed to lose weight with a low fat diet and is currently healthy, could start experimenting with days when more macronutrients come from fat; such experiments would be carried randomly, to prevent the body from habituation (to the diet), thus making it more prepared in 'handling' unpredictable and different dietary situations.

Similarly, a person who followed a ketogenic diet could experiment with high-carb days, challenging the body in its ability to become more metabolically flexible. I used to be very much against this because in my head I used to think that if I do it, I'll lose some self-imposed 'keto-adapted' status. Simplistic and reductionist explanations from other people have ingrained such thoughts into my mind. It took a lot of time until I started questioning and subjecting those beliefs to scrutiny.

My point is that even though one may want be fairly consistent with a certain type of diet, to increase the flexibility of one's metabolic engine, one should experiment with different inputs, administered with a certain frequency. Simply put, if you enjoy your low-fat diet or your high-fat diet, I'm not telling you to bash it. I'm saying that if you're healthy, you could try subjecting your body to unpredictable dietary inputs from time to time; it may support your long term adherence and you may be surprised of the results.

For a few years, I completely removed gluten from my diet, along with foods that are higher in carbohydrates. In retrospect, I embraced this limiting belief without too much questioning. As I became more aware of our innate biases, in particular to this situation, I said to my self: Hey, why not try a piece of rye bread and see what happens? Will my body go crazy?

It did not. Nothing happened actually. I did not experience negative short-term effects. Then I started experimenting with other foodstuff (that I had been avoiding), while keeping some of my core nutrition in place. A baked potato here, after gym, some more rye bread there, a piece of fruit... They all seem to fit in my current, very dynamic, nutrition protocol.

Similarly, I moved away from a self-imposed phobia of 'toxins'. I moved away from the non-GMO, organic, grass-fed non-sense. While I try to focus on consuming whole foods from all dietary *spectra*, I will allow dietary perturbations here and there, for the sake of challenging my system. You can think of dietary perturbations as: high-fructose corn syrup, food additives and preservatives, common allergens, added sugar, and many other ingredients that come in packaged, processed foods, and not only. In fact, some recent research proposes gradual exposure to and consumption of peanuts as treatment for people with peanut allergies. The immune system is untrained, weakened, and unchallenged when you remove all perturbations.

These perturbations should challenge and stress my body, making it more prepared to handle subsequent and possibly more severe challenges (if that ever becomes the case). Would I recommend this to an unhealthy person? Of course not! Get yourself back on track first; maybe thereafter you could try challenging your body for the sake of growing healthier; otherwise this may do you no good.

Other dietary stressors that one could use and which I randomly use come from plant toxins, phytochemicals and phytonutrients. The super-family of CYP450 (Cytochrome P450) proteins, in their effort to handle these stressors, may trigger endogenous mechanisms (adaptive responses) to increase body's resilience.

Do I believe in detox fads, juicing or cleansing? Nope, not at the moment. I think that the best detoxification machineries are already inside us (liver, kidneys, skin, and other excretory organs). This does not mean that green juices are not supportive of health. But this is far from the outrageous 'curing' claims you are being confronted with everyday, such as: 'cure cancer with food', 'fight cancer with juice', 'make yourself 10 years younger juicing', and so on.

Supplementation with or exposure to plant toxins is a strategy that I imply randomly and selectively. Other than that, I currently have a few unordinary items that I use in my diet, to increase my fiber intake, such as: psyllium husk, hemp husk, and apple pectin.

They come on top of a diet abundant in vegetables and plant foods. Removing the very top layer of grapefruits and lemons and blending them to obtain a thick paste that I would use in a mix with cold water throughout the day is another strategy.

There are days when I consume higher carbs, days of lower carbs, days of underfeeding and caloric restriction, days of overfeeding, days of dietary ketosis, and days of complete fasting. My prolonged fasts are infrequent and random. It is all contextual and very dynamic.

Even though I currently and for the last two years have been doing intermittent fasting (18-22 hours of fasting), there have been periods of 3-4 weeks (in these past years) when I increased my feeding window to 12 hours a day. I think that intermittent fasting and prolonged fasting can aid health, which is why I have kept them in my repertoire. I try to break from them every now and then. Breaking allows for resensitization to these stimuli.

I adopt a similar, cyclical and random approach to alcohol and caffeine intake. While I mostly never consume more than 2 glasses of wine at once, there have been periods when I had this 'amount' every few days. There have been periods when I had it less frequently, such as once or twice a week, and there have been periods of complete abstinence. Anecdotally, my sleep seems to be much better when alcohol is absent from my system.

Similarly, I cycle through periods of higher caffeine intake (a few cups a day) and periods with low caffeine intake, when I consume decaffeinated coffee.

As for other aspects of my life:

I have numerous strategies for weight-lifting. I always play with variables such as: frequency, load, and volume, while I almost always try to keep the intensity high and a progressive overload approach.

Sometimes, I go to the gym at odd hours. I try to prevent my body from getting used to working out only at certain hours of the day or certain days of the week. Sometimes, I'm in the gym for 5-7 days/week, while other times I go there once or twice a week. When I take time off from lifting for a few weeks, I focus on short-burst high-intensity training.

I randomize cold exposure: sometimes getting into a very cold shower immediately after a workout (I don't recommend doing this), sometimes taking 2-3 cold showers per day, often taking cold and ice-baths. But cold is not the norm as it used to be. I also take hot showers, warm baths, and get into the infra-red sauna every now and then.

Such randomness, apparent lack of order, and unpredictability in my life comes with effort. One can see how easy it may be to: go to the gym 3 times a week, do the same exercises, eat the same food, follow the same diet, and do everything habitually. My current strategy appears to be the opposite because I do not think that one can grow from comfortable and highly predictable customs.

Exposing my body to stressors and to unpredictability may be a good way to have it always be prepared to facing harder challenges. My strategies require getting comfortable with discomfort, getting comfortable with facing the unpredictable, not knowing that you might change your mind the very next second. Here's an example:

I go to the gym and lift weights for an hour. While lifting, I could envision the rest of my day: take a hot shower, go home and eat, work, meet with friends and family. It looks good on paper. Instead, once I finish lifting, I jump into a very cold shower for 10 minutes, then I skip eating until later in the day and sometimes even later at night.

It is very uncomfortable; however, satisfaction always seems to come after the fact.

Please understand, cold exposure, if done 'correctly', should make one feel miserable - shivering for the next few hours. Any physiologic stressor should create discomfort, unease, and unpleasantness for the short term.

As soon as you stop responding to a stressor, you might have to change one or more of the variables: higher dose, frequency, or duration, or a strategy of resensitization - deprivation from the stressor.

Getting all of this right is very challenging. One could easily slide into chronic stress, which will most likely be detrimental. Additionally, recovery is necessary for growth from the action of stressors; such recovery and complete deprivation of exposure can serve as resensitization, allowing one to restart exposure to the stressor at a later time and a much lower dose, frequency, and duration of exposure.

I am implying a cyclical approach to stressors: progressively adapting to, followed by resensitization, recovery and growth.

One cannot use stressors without feeling uncomfortable, uneased, and, possibly, miserable. Whether it's a physiologic stressor (dietary stress, plant toxins and phytochemicals, oxidants, toxic chemicals, food deprivation, cold and heat exposure, hypergravity, hypoxia, etc) or cognitive stressors that create mental discomfort, they all imply deliberately subjecting oneself to discomfort.

There is no short-circuiting the process, no hack for this. In my current philosophy, antifragility is forged through the fire of perturbing stress.

This book was about stress and adaptation, physiologic and psychologic perturbations, finding the right dose, frequency and duration at which a stressor can be beneficial. This book was also an overview of stressors, from a molecular to a whole system's perspective. While I may have alluded to concepts such as hormesis here and there, I currently do not think that one needs to use such words to understand stress, adaptation and dose-response relationships.

While the book may be more accessible to an audience familiar with biological terminology, it is my hope that my personal examples and anecdotes may have made it available to less technical readers as well. My personal examples may be relevant to many readers, but I do not intend to serve them as guide, especially in light of their unpredictable, dynamic and ever changing nature.

In my ending thought, I hope that this book revealed to you a facet of stressors, stress and adaptation, that will serve for the betterment of your life.

Acknowledgements

How could this have been possible were it not for the amazing scientists, researchers, and leading individuals who have created and contributed to the field? How could this book have existed were it not for Hans Selye and his decades long exploration of stress physiology, for Irina Milisav and her contribution to molecular and cellular adaptive stress responses, for the works of researchers and door openers such as Mark P. Mattson of the NIA, Rattan Suresh, Edward Calabrese, Martha Stark and other contemporary names who are actively contributing to the field? How can I not mention Nassim Taleb for influencing my world view with his perspectives on randomness and anti-fragility?

I would like to thank them, the researchers, scientists and authors you find in the bibliography, and other people who have influenced me in a direct or indirect way.

I would like to thank my friend Red O'Laughlin for providing valuable feedback and for assisting with the editing. I appreciate you Red!

Last, but not least, I would like to thank my family, whom unquestionably put up with and accepted my caprices, stubbornness and the lack of time I often invoked when my presence was needed or desired.

Stress and Adaptation in Physiology

Bibliography

1. McGing, B. C. (1986). *The Foreign Policy of Mithridates VI Eupator, King of Pontus* (Vol. 89). Brill.

2. Mattson, M. P., & Calabrese, E. J. (Eds.). (2009). *Hormesis: a revolution in biology, toxicology and medicine.* Springer Science & Business Media.

3. Sánchez, F. G., & Rial, B. R. (2005). Orthorexia nervosa. A new eating behavior disorder?. *Actas Esp Psiquiatr, 33*(1), 66-68.

4. Becker, T. (2010). Cold showers. Retrieved from http://gettingstronger.org/2010/03/cold-showers/

5. Vlad, C. (2013). The Icy-Cold Experiment. Retrieved from http://cristivlad.com/icy-cold-experiment/

6. Stewart, W. K., & Fleming, L. W. (1973). Features of a successful therapeutic fast of 382 days' duration. *Postgraduate medical journal, 49*(569), 203-209.

7. Homeostasis. (2016). *Collins English Dictionary - Complete & Unabridged 10th Edition.* Retrieved from http://dictionary.refcrence.com/browse/homeostasis

8. Wikipedia (2016). Homeostasis. Retrieved from https://en.wikipedia.org/wiki/Homeostasis

9. Merriam Webster (2016). Homeopathy. Retrieved from http://www.merriam-webster.com/dictionary/homeopathy

10. The Society of Homeopaths (2016). About Homeopathy. Retrieved from http://www.homeopathy-soh.org/about-homeopathy

11. Tuomela, R. (1987). Science, protoscience, and pseudoscience. In *Rational Changes in Science* (pp. 83-101). Springer Netherlands.

12. Smith, K. (2012). Homeopathy is unscientific and unethical. *Bioethics, 26*(9), 508-512.

13. Baran, G. R., Kiani, M. F., & Samuel, S. P. (2014). Science, Pseudoscience, and Not Science: How Do They Differ?. In *Healthcare and Biomedical Technology in the 21st Century* (pp. 19-57). Springer New York.

14. Pigliucci, M., & Boudry, M. (Eds.). (2013). *Philosophy of pseudoscience: reconsidering the demarcation problem*. University of Chicago Press.

15. Ernst, E. (2002). A systematic review of systematic reviews of homeopathy. *British journal of clinical pharmacology, 54*(6), 577-582.

16. Shang, A., Huwiler-Müntener, K., Nartey, L., Jüni, P., Dörig, S., Sterne, J. A., ... & Egger, M. (2005). Are the clinical effects of homoeopathy placebo effects? Comparative study of placebo-controlled trials of homoeopathy and allopathy. *The Lancet, 366*(9487), 726-732.

17. U.K. Parliament (2010). Evidence Check 2: Homeopathy: Science and Technology Committee. Retrieved from http://www.publications.parliament.uk/pa/cm200910/cmselect/cmsctech/45/4504.htm

18. Mattson, M. P. (2016). Full Curriculum Vitae - Mark P. Mattson - 2014. Retrieved from http://neuroscience.jhu.edu/uploads/publications/Mattson_M/MattsonFullCV_January_2014.doc

19. Mattson, M. P. (2016). Author Mark P. Mattson. Retrieved from
https://scholar.google.ro/citations?user=N3ObarMAAAAJ&hl=en

20. Calabrese, E. J. (2016). Edward J. Calabrese - Faculty Page. Retrieved from
https://www.umass.edu/sphhs/person/faculty/edward-j-calabrese

21. Calabrese, E. J. (2016). Full Curriculum Vitae - Edward J. Calabrese - 2013. Retrieved from
https://www.umass.edu/sphhs/sites/default/files/CV_Calabrese_Aug2013.pdf

22. Cato Institute (2016). Cato's Mission. Retrieved from
http://www.cato.org/mission

23. Rattan, S. (2016). Research and Review Articles. Retrieved from http://sureshrattan.com/category/publications/c35-research-papers/

24. NIH Office of Science Education (2016). Dose-Response Relationships. Retrieved from
https://science.education.nih.gov/supplements/nih2/chemicals/guide/pdfs/lesson3.pdf

25. Robertson, A., Allen, J., Laney, R., & Curnow, A. (2013). The cellular and molecular carcinogenic effects of radon exposure: a review. *International journal of molecular sciences*, 14(7), 14024-14063.

26. Cohen, B. L. (1995). Test of the linear-no threshold theory of radiation carcinogenesis for inhaled radon decay products. *Health Physics*, 68(2), 157-174.

27. Yarris, L. (2011). New Take on Impacts of Low Dose Radiation. Retrieved from http://newscenter.lbl.gov/2011/12/20/low-dose-radiation/

28. Olipitz, W., Wiktor-Brown, D., Shuga, J., Pang, B., McFaline, J., Lonkar, P., ... & Dedon, P. C. (2012). Integrated molecular analysis indicates undetectable change in DNA damage in mice after continuous irradiation at~ 400-fold natural background radiation. *Environmental health perspectives, 120*(8), 1130.

29. Calabrese, E. J. (2011). Muller's Nobel lecture on dose–response for ionizing radiation: ideology or science?. *Archives of toxicology, 85*(12), 1495-1498.

30. Tubiana, M., & Aurengo, A. (2006). Dose–effect relationship and estimation of the carcinogenic effects of low doses of ionising radiation: the Joint Report of the Académie des Sciences (Paris) and of the Académie Nationale de Médecine. *International Journal of Low Radiation, 2*(3-4), 135-153.

31. Health Physics Society (2010). Radiation Risk in Perspective. Retrieved from http://hps.org/documents/risk_ps010-2.pdf

32. RationalWiki (2016). Linear No Threshold. Retrieved from http://rationalwiki.org/wiki/Linear_no-threshold

33. Stannered (2016). Wikimedia Commons. Retrieved from https://en.wikipedia.org/wiki/Hormesis

34. Tubiana, M., Feinendegen, L. E., Yang, C., & Kaminski, J. M. (2009). The linear no-threshold relationship is inconsistent with radiation biologic and experimental data 1. *Radiology, 251*(1), 13-22.

35. Vandenberg, L. N., Colborn, T., Hayes, T. B., Heindel, J. J., Jacobs Jr, D. R., Lee, D. H., ... & Zoeller, R. T. (2012). Hormones

and endocrine-disrupting chemicals: low-dose effects and nonmonotonic dose responses. *Endocrine reviews, 33*(3), 378-455.

36. Mattson, M. P. (2015). Toxic Chemicals in Fruits and Vegetables Are What Give Them Their Health Benefits. *Scientific American,* Vol. 313(1).

37. Vasquez, A. (2004). *Integrative Orthopedics: Concepts, Algorithms, and Therapeutics: the Art of Creating Wellness While Effectively Managing Acute and Chronic Musculoskeletal Disorders.* Natural Health Consulting Corporation.

38. Texel, S. J., & Mattson, M. P. (2011). Impaired adaptive cellular responses to oxidative stress and the pathogenesis of Alzheimer's disease. *Antioxidants & redox signaling, 14*(8), 1519-1534.

39. Calabrese, E. J. (2015). Hormesis: principles and applications. *Homeopathy, 104*(2), 69-82.

40. Kitchin, K. T., & Drane, J. W. (2005). A critique of the use of hormesis in risk assessment. *Human & experimental toxicology, 24*(5), 249-253.

41. Thayer, K. A., Melnick, R., Burns, K., Davis, D., & Huff, J. (2005). Fundamental flaws of hormesis for public health decisions. *Environmental health perspectives,* 1271-1276.

42. Szabo, S., Tache, Y., & Somogyi, A. (2012). The legacy of Hans Selye and the origins of stress research: a retrospective 75 years after his landmark brief "letter" to the editor# of nature. *Stress, 15*(5), 472-478.

43. Selye, H. (1936). A syndrome produced by diverse nocuous agents. *Nature, 138*(3479), 32.

44. Selye, H. (2013). *Stress in health and disease*. Butterworth-Heinemann.

45. Calabrese, E. J., Bachmann, K. A., Bailer, A. J., Bolger, P. M., Borak, J., Cai, L., ... & Cook, R. R. (2007). Biological stress response terminology: integrating the concepts of adaptive response and preconditioning stress within a hormetic dose–response framework. *Toxicology and applied pharmacology, 222*(1), 122-128.

46. Oken, B. S., Chamine, I., & Wakeland, W. (2015). A systems approach to stress, stressors and resilience in humans. *Behavioural brain research, 282*, 144-154.

47. Davies, K. J. (2016). Adaptive homeostasis. *Molecular aspects of medicine, 49*, 1-7.

48. Guyton, A. C., & Hall, J. E. (1991). *Textbook of Medical Physiology*. Saunders, Philadelphia, PA.

49. Timiras, P. & Chetty, S. (2008). MCB 135k: Physiology of the Aging Process. Retrieved from http://mcb.berkeley.edu/courses/mcb135k/allostasis.html

50. Schulkin, J. (2004). *Allostasis, homeostasis, and the costs of physiological adaptation*. Cambridge University Press.

51. Suresh, R. & Le Bourg, E. (2014). *Hormesis in health and disease*. CRC Press.

52. Vinten-Johansen, J., Yellon, D. M., & Opie, L. H. (2005). Postconditioning A Simple, Clinically Applicable Procedure to Improve Revascularization in Acute Myocardial Infarction. *Circulation, 112*(14), 2085-2088.

53. Demirovic, D., de Toda, I. M., & Rattan, S. (2014). Molecular stress response pathways as the basis of hormesis. In *Hormesis in Health and Disease*. CRC Press LLC.

54. Choi, A. M., Ryter, S. W., & Levine, B. (2013). Autophagy in human health and disease. *New England Journal of Medicine, 368*(7), 651-662.

55. Scherz-Shouval, R., & Elazar, Z. (2011). Regulation of autophagy by ROS: physiology and pathology. *Trends in biochemical sciences, 36*(1), 30-38.

56. Yang, Z., & Klionsky, D. J. (2010). Eaten alive: a history of macroautophagy. *Nature cell biology, 12*(9), 814-822.

57. Sack, M. N., & Finkel, T. (2012). Mitochondrial metabolism, sirtuins, and aging. *Cold Spring Harbor perspectives in biology, 4*(12), a013102.

58. Jackson, S. P., & Bartek, J. (2009). The DNA-damage response in human biology and disease. *Nature, 461*(7267), 1071-1078.

59. Zhang, H., Ryu, D., Wu, Y., Gariani, K., Wang, X., Luan, P., ... & Schoonjans, K. (2016). NAD+ repletion improves mitochondrial and stem cell function and enhances life span in mice. *Science*, aaf2693.

60. Crawford, D. R., & Davies, K. J. (1994). Adaptive response and oxidative stress. *Environmental health perspectives, 102*(Suppl 10), 25.

61. Milisav, I. (2011). Cellular stress responses. *Advances in Regenerative Medicine*, 215-232.

62. Milisav, I., Poljsak, B., & Šuput, D. (2012). Adaptive response, evidence of cross-resistance and its potential clinical use. *International journal of molecular sciences, 13*(9), 10771-10806.

63. Hadley, C. (2003). What doesn't kill you makes you stronger. *EMBO reports, 4*(10), 924-926.

64. Mattson, M. P. (2008). Hormesis and disease resistance: activation of cellular stress response pathways. *Human & experimental toxicology, 27*(2), 155-162.

65. Schoenfeld, B. (2016). *Strong & Sculpted*. Human Kinetics.

66. Peterson, M. D., Rhea, M. R., & Alvar, B. A. (2004). Maximizing strength development in athletes: a meta-analysis to determine the dose-response relationship. *The Journal of Strength & Conditioning Research, 18*(2), 377-382.

67. Lesinski, M., Prieske, O., & Granacher, U. (2016). Effects and dose–response relationships of resistance training on physical performance in youth athletes: a systematic review and meta-analysis. *British journal of sports medicine*, bjsports-2015.

68. Rhea, M. R., Alvar, B. A., Burkett, L. N., & Ball, S. D. (2003). A meta-analysis to determine the dose response for strength development. *Medicine and science in sports and exercise, 35*(3), 456-464.

69. de Morton, N. A. (2009). The PEDro scale is a valid measure of the methodological quality of clinical trials: a demographic study. *Australian Journal of Physiotherapy, 55*(2), 129-133.

70. Sidney University (2016). PEDro Scale. Retrieved from http://www.pedro.org.au/english/downloads/pedro-scale/

71. Schoenfeld, B. J. (2010). The mechanisms of muscle hypertrophy and their application to resistance training. *The Journal of Strength & Conditioning Research, 24*(10), 2857-2872.

72. Toigo, M., & Boutellier, U. (2006). New fundamental resistance exercise determinants of molecular and cellular muscle adaptations. *European journal of applied physiology, 97*(6), 643-663.

73. Rennie, M. J., Wackerhage, H., Spangenburg, E. E., & Booth, F. W. (2004). Control of the size of the human muscle mass. *Annu. Rev. Physiol., 66*, 799-828.

74. Crewther, B., Cronin, J., & Keogh, J. (2006). Possible stimuli for strength and power adaptation. Sports medicine, 36(3), 215-238.

75. Schoenfeld, B. (2011). The use of specialized training techniques to maximize muscle hypertrophy. Strength & Conditioning Journal, 33(4), 60-65.

76. Barton, P. (2015). Muscles: Actions, Movements, and Terminology. Retrieved from http://slideplayer.com/slide/4746005/

77. Fleck, S. (2011). Non-linear periodization for general fitness & athletes. *Journal of human kinetics, 29*(Special Issue), 41-45.

78. Schoenfeld, B. J., Contreras, B., Ogborn, D., Galpin, A., Krieger, J., & Sonmez, G. T. (2016). Effects of Varied Versus Constant Loading Zones on Muscular Adaptations in Trained Men. *International journal of sports medicine, 37*(06), 442-447.

79. Peake, J. M., Markworth, J. F., Nosaka, K., Raastad, T., Wadley, G. D., & Coffey, V. G. (2015). Modulating exercise-induced hormesis: does less equal more?. *Journal of Applied Physiology, 119*(3), 172-189.

80. Gradari, S., Pallé, A., McGreevy, K. R., Fontán-Lozano, Á., & Trejo, J. L. (2016). Can Exercise Make You Smarter, Happier, and Have More Neurons? A Hormetic Perspective. *Frontiers in neuroscience, 10*.

81. Volek, J. S., Freidenreich, D. J., Saenz, C., Kunces, L. J., Creighton, B. C., Bartley, J. M., ... & Lee, E. C. (2016). Metabolic characteristics of keto-adapted ultra-endurance runners. *Metabolism, 65*(3), 100-110.

82. Vandereycken, W. (2011). Media hype, diagnostic fad or genuine disorder? Professionals' opinions about night eating syndrome, orthorexia, muscle dysmorphia, and emetophobia. *Eating disorders, 19*(2), 145-155.

83. Bratman, S. (2014). What is Orthorexia? Retrieved from http://www.orthorexia.com/what-is-orthorexia/

84. Bartrina, J. A. (2007). [Orthorexia or when a healthy diet becomes an obsession]. *Archivos latinoamericanos de nutricion, 57*(4), 313-315.

85. Koven, N. S., & Abry, A. W. (2015). The clinical basis of orthorexia nervosa: emerging perspectives. *Neuropsychiatric Disease & Treatment, 11*.

86. Donini, L. M., Marsili, D., Graziani, M. P., Imbriale, M., & Cannella, C. (2004). Orthorexia nervosa: a preliminary study with a proposal for diagnosis and an attempt to measure the dimension of the phenomenon. *Eating and Weight Disorders-Studies on Anorexia, Bulimia and Obesity, 9*(2), 151-157.

87. Pall, M. L., & Levine, S. (2015). Nrf2, a master regulator of detoxification and also antioxidant, anti-inflammatory and other cytoprotective mechanisms, is raised by health promoting factors. *Sheng Li Xue Bao, 67*(1), 1-18.

88. Speciale, A., Chirafisi, J., Saija, A., & Cimino, F. (2011). Nutritional antioxidants and adaptive cell responses: an update. *Current molecular medicine, 11*(9), 770-789.

89. Birringer, M. (2011). Hormetics: dietary triggers of an adaptive stress response. *Pharmaceutical research, 28*(11), 2680-2694.

90. Hooper, P. L., Hooper, P. L., Tytell, M., & Vígh, L. (2010). Xenohormesis: health benefits from an eon of plant stress response evolution. *Cell Stress and Chaperones, 15*(6), 761-770.

91. Son, T. G., Camandola, S., & Mattson, M. P. (2008). Hormetic dietary phytochemicals. *Neuromolecular medicine, 10*(4), 236-246.

92. Howitz, K. T., & Sinclair, D. A. (2008). Xenohormesis: sensing the chemical cues of other species. *Cell, 133*(3), 387-391.

93. Morris, B. J. (2008). How xenohormetic compounds confer health benefits. In *Mild Stress and Healthy Aging* (pp. 115-138). Springer Netherlands.

94. World Health Organization (2015). Global Information System on Alcohol and Health. Retrieved from http://www.who.int/gho/alcohol/en/

95. Martin, B., Ji, S., White, C. M., Maudsley, S., & Mattson, M. P. (2010). Dietary Energy Intake, Hormesis, and Health. In *Hormesis* (pp. 123-137). Humana Press.

96. Martin, B., Mattson, M. P., & Maudsley, S. (2006). Caloric restriction and intermittent fasting: two potential diets for successful brain aging. *Ageing research reviews, 5*(3), 332-353.

97. Lam, Y. Y., & Ravussin, E. (2014). 5 Periodic Fasting. *Hormesis in Health and Disease, 79*.

98. Testa, G., Biasi, F., Poli, G., & Chiarpotto, E. (2014). Calorie restriction and dietary restriction mimetics: a strategy for improving healthy aging and longevity. Current pharmaceutical design, 20(18), 2950-2977.

99. Scapagnini, G., Davinelli, S., Fortunati, N. A., Zella, D., & Vitale, M. (2014). Thermal hydrotherapy as adaptive stress response: hormetic significance, mechanisms, and therapeutic implications.

100. Stocks, J. M., Taylor, N. A., Tipton, M. J., & Greenleaf, J. E. (2004). Human physiological responses to cold exposure. *Aviation, space, and environmental medicine, 75(5),* 444-457.

101. Kaciuba-Uscilko, H., & Greenleaf, J. E. (1989). Acclimatization to cold in humans.

102. Leppäluoto, J., Pääkkönen, T., Korhonen, I., & Hassi, J. (2005). Pituitary and autonomic responses to cold exposures in man. *Acta physiologica scandinavica, 184(4),* 255-264.

103. Ostrowski, K., Rohde, T., Asp, S., Schjerling, P., & Pedersen, B. K. (1999). Pro-and anti-inflammatory cytokine balance in strenuous exercise in humans. *The Journal of physiology, 515(1),* 287-291.

104. Dr. Rhonda Patrick (2016). Cold Stress Report. Retrieved from http://foundmyfitness.com/?sendme=cold-stress

105. Leppäluoto, J., Westerlund, T., Huttunen, P., Oksa, J., Smolander, J., Dugué, B., & Mikkelsson, M. (2008). Effects of long-term whole-body cold exposures on plasma concentrations of ACTH, beta-endorphin, cortisol, catecholamines and cytokines in healthy females. *Scandinavian journal of clinical and laboratory investigation, 68(2),* 145-153.

106. Lubkowska, A., Dołęgowska, B., & Szyguła, Z. (2012). Whole-body cryostimulation-potential beneficial treatment for improving antioxidant capacity in healthy men-significance of the number of sessions. *Plos one, 7(10)*, e46352.

107. Fukai, T., & Ushio-Fukai, M. (2011). Superoxide dismutases: role in redox signaling, vascular function, and diseases. *Antioxidants & redox signaling, 15(6)*, 1583-1606.

108. Vaiserman, A. (2014). 7 Radiation Exposure. *Hormesis in Health and Disease*, 107.

109. Karam, P. A., & Leslie, S. A. (1999). Calculations of background beta-gamma radiation dose through geologic time. *Health physics, 77(6)*, 662-667.

110. Russo, G. L., Tedesco, I., Russo, M., Cioppa, A., Andreassi, M. G., & Picano, E. (2012). Cellular adaptive response to chronic radiation exposure in interventional cardiologists. *European heart journal, 33(3)*, 408-414.

111. Feinendegen, L. E., Pollycove, M., & Neumann, R. D. (2007). Whole-body responses to low-level radiation exposure: new concepts in mammalian radiobiology. *Experimental hematology, 35(4)*, 37-46.

112. Feinendegen, L. E. (2005). Evidence for beneficial low level radiation effects and radiation hormesis. *The British journal of radiology*.

113. Scott, B. R., & Di Palma, J. (2007). Sparsely ionizing diagnostic and natural background radiations are likely preventing cancer and other genomic-instability-associated diseases. *Dose-Response, 5(3)*, dose-response.

114. Scott, B. R., Haque, M., & Di Palma, J. (2007). Biological basis for radiation hormesis in mammalian cellular communities. *International Journal of Low Radiation, 4*(1), 1-16.

115. Frigerio, N. A., & Stowe, R. S. (1976). Carcinogenic and genetic hazard from background radiation. In *Biological and environmental effects of low-level radiation.*

116. Feinendegen, L. F., & Pollycove, M. (2001). Biologic responses to low doses of ionizing radiation: Detriment versus hormesis--part 1. Dose responses of cells and tissues. *The Journal of Nuclear Medicine, 42*(7), N17.

117. Pollycove, M., & Feinendegen, L. E. (2003). Radiation-induced versus endogenous DNA damage: possible effect of inducible protective responses in mitigating endogenous damage. *Human & experimental toxicology, 22*(6), 290-306.

118. Feinendegen, L. E., Pollycove, M., & Sondhaus, C. A. (2004). Responses to low doses of ionizing radiation in biological systems. *Nonlinearity in biology, toxicology, medicine, 2*(3), 15401420490507431.

119. Jargin, S. V. (2012). Hormesis and radiation safety norms. *Human & experimental toxicology, 31*(7), 671-675.

120. Duan, P., Quan, C., Hu, C., Zhang, J., Xie, F., Hu, X., ... & Liu, C. (2015). Nonlinear dose–response relationship between radon exposure and the risk of lung cancer: evidence from a meta-analysis of published observational studies. *European Journal of Cancer Prevention, 24*(4), 267-277.

121. Tang, F. R., & Loke, W. K. (2015). Molecular mechanisms of low dose ionizing radiation-induced hormesis, adaptive responses, radioresistance, bystander effects, and genomic instability. *International journal of radiation biology, 91*(1), 13-27.

122. Nageswari, K. (2015). Mobile Phone Radiation: Physiological & Pathophysiologcal Considerations.

123. Novella, S. (2016). Still No Association of Cell Phones and Brain Cancer. Retrieved from http://theness.com/neurologicablog/index.php/still-no-association-of-cell-phones-and-brain-cancer/

124. SEER.Cancer.Gov (2016). Cancer of the Brain and other Nervous System. SEER Stat Fact Sheet. Retrieved from http://seer.cancer.gov/statfacts/html/brain.html

125. Schlebusch, C. M., Gattepaille, L. M., Engström, K., Vahter, M., Jakobsson, M., & Broberg, K. (2015). Human adaptation to arsenic-rich environments. *Molecular biology and evolution, 32*(6), 1544-1555.

126. Brookshire, B. (2015). Arsenic Spurs Adaptation in Argentinean Villagers. Retrieved from https://www.sciencenews.org/blog/science-ticker/arsenic-spurs-adaptation-argentinian-villagers

127. Schlebusch, C. M., Lewis Jr, C. M., Vahter, M., Engström, K., Tito, R. Y., Obregón-Tito, A. J., ... & Concha, G. (2013). Possible positive selection for an arsenic-protective haplotype in humans. *Environmental Health Perspectives (Online), 121*(1), 53.

128. Pierce, B. L., Kibriya, M. G., Tong, L., Jasmine, F., Argos, M., Roy, S., ... & Ahmed, A. (2012). Genome-wide association study identifies chromosome 10q24. 32 variants associated with arsenic metabolism and toxicity phenotypes in Bangladesh. *PLoS Genet, 8*(2), e1002522.

129. Ioannidis, J. P. (2005). Why most published research findings are false. *PLoS Med, 2*(8), e124.

130. Lin, K., Hsin, H., Libina, N., & Kenyon, C. (2001). Regulation of the Caenorhabditis elegans longevity protein DAF-16 by insulin/IGF-1 and germline signaling. *Nature genetics, 28*(2), 139-145.

131. Rattan, S. I. (2008). Hormesis in aging. *Ageing research reviews, 7*(1), 63-78.

132. Rattan, S. I. (2007). Homeostasis, homeodynamics, and aging. *Encyclopedia of Gerontology. 2nd edition ed. UK: Elsevier Inc,* 696-9.

133. Leslie, M. (2005). How can we use moderate stresses to fortify humans and slow aging?. *Science's SAGE KE, 2005*(26), nf49.

134. Radak, Z., Chung, H. Y., Koltai, E., Taylor, A. W., & Goto, S. (2008). Exercise, oxidative stress and hormesis. *Ageing research reviews, 7*(1), 34-42.

135. Kyriazis, M. (2010). Nonlinear stimulation and hormesis in human aging: practical examples and action mechanisms. *Rejuvenation research, 13*(4), 445-452.

136. Chadwick, W., & Maudsley, S. (2010). The devil is in the dose: complexity of receptor systems and responses. In *Hormesis* (pp. 95-108). Humana Press.

137. Stark, M. (2014). Optimal Stress, Psychological Resilience, and the Sandpile Model. In S. I. Rattan, & É. Le Bourg (Eds.), *Hormesis in Health and Disease* (pp. 199-222). CRC Press.

138. Baldwin, J. (1961). Nobody Knows My Name: A Letter from the South. *Nobody Knows My Name: More Notes of a Native Son,* 98-116.

139. Carver, C. S. (1998). Resilience and thriving: Issues, models, and linkages. *Journal of social issues, 54*(2), 245-266.

140. Greco, V., & Roger, D. (2003). Uncertainty, stress, and health. *Personality and Individual differences, 34*(6), 1057-1068.

141. Geddes, L. (2012). Anti-fragile: the new power word. *New Scientist, 216*(2891), 30-31.

142. Taleb, N. N. (2012). *Antifragile: how to live in a world we don't understand* (Vol. 3). London: Allen Lane.

143. Taleb, N. N. (2007). *The black swan: The impact of the highly improbable*. Random house.

144. Taleb, N. N. (2012). *Antifragile: Things that gain from disorder* (Vol. 3). Random House Incorporated.

145. Thomas, G. (2013). Hormesis vs. Leviathan. Accessed at http://redstateeclectic.typepad.com/redstate_commentary/2013/03/hormesis-versus-leviathan.html

Stress and Adaptation in Physiology

Other Works from the same Author

1. Ketone Power - Superfuel for Optimal Mental Health and Ultimate Physical Performance

2. T-(Rx) - The Testosterone Protocol - On Achieving True Male Status

3. Periodic Fasting - Repair your DNA, Grow Younger, and Learn to Appreciate your Food

4. Urban Escape - A Digital Entrepreneur's Travel Guide for New York City

5. Persistent Fat Loss - Combining Ketosis and Intermittent Fasting for Year-Round Fitness

6. Mastering Udemy - How I Published my First Online Course

More information and a detailed bio of the author at:
http://cristivlad.com

www.ingramcontent.com/pod-product-compliance
Lightning Source LLC
Chambersburg PA
CBHW021424170526
45164CB00001B/85